Contents

The Peer Appraisal Handbook for General Practitioners

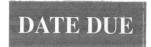
Hilary Haman

Sally Irvine

and Di Jelley

Foreword by

Dame Lesley Southgate

Radcliffe Medical Press

© 2001 Hilary Haman, Sally Irvine and Di Jelley

Radcliffe Medical Press Ltd
18 Marcham Road, Abingdon, Oxon OX14 1AA

British Library Cataloguing in Publication Data

A catalogue record for this book is available from the British Library.

ISBN 1 85775 570 7

Typeset by Aarontype Limited, Easton, Bristol
Printed and bound by TJ International Ltd, Padstow, Cornwall

Foreword

We are frequently told that the rate of change in medicine has never been greater. This is coupled with the development of modern relationships between doctors and patients characterised by partnership rather than paternalism and by explicit expectations of a doctor's competence and communication. The same themes are presently played out in the relationship between society and the profession, usually mediated through government and the media. But while accountability is to be welcomed whole-heartedly, the climate within which it manifests is of prime importance.

This book marks a contribution to a climate of encouragement, reward and facilitation. In so doing it does not provide an escape route for poor practice, but rather a rigorous and practical approach to supporting all practitioners to do a good job, and gain satisfaction while doing so.

Although the handbook includes detailed and sensible advice on how to carry out peer appraisal, it is also founded on explicit values. It takes the General Medical Council's guidance for all doctors, elaborated as *Good Medical Practice for General Practitioners*, as its template and uses best practice from industry and medical practice to enable individuals to be appraised in every aspect by peers. The relationships to revalidation and managerial job review are made clear, as is the foundation principle that this is a formative activity. By using this approach, which builds trust, relationships, teams and practices, and which explicitly avoids collusion with poor standards, the fabric of the practice and the confidence of the individual doctor will be strengthened.

Most of the documented improvements in general practice over the last 20 years have been achieved by supporting each other without being afraid to give and receive feedback from peers, colleagues and patients. In this handbook the reader will find an activity framed in the best tradition of general practice, not least the commitment to quality improvement, self-appraisal and a focus on better healthcare for patients.

Dame Lesley Southgate
Professor of Primary Care and Medical Education,
RFUC Medical School
President, Royal College of General Practitioners
February 2001

About the authors

Hilary Haman has over 20 years' experience in personnel management including running human resource departments in both the public and private sectors. Hilary first became professionally involved in primary healthcare in 1986 when she joined the Royal College of General Practitioners in London as head of personnel.

Since 1990 she has worked as an independent management consultant mainly in general practice although she has other clients in the private, public and voluntary sectors. Her work encompasses providing advice on personnel issues, including the application of employment law, designing and running management development courses and, with Sally Irvine as Haman and Irvine Associates (HIA), undertaking organisational reviews of individual practices and developing management tools for general practice.

Throughout her career Hilary has been involved in, and led on, designing, introducing and evaluating appraisal schemes for the different organisations in which she has worked. In 1992, Hilary designed and delivered the first residential performance appraisal course held at the RCGP for members and practice managers. It is this course, through several evolutions, which she now delivers, with Sally Irvine, across the country and which informed the content of this handbook.

Hilary Haman is a Fellow of the Chartered Institute of Personnel and Development and a Member of the Institute of Healthcare Management. She writes extensively on management and personnel issues within primary care and lives in Cardiff with her husband, David, and son, Alexander.

Sally Irvine has a wide understanding and knowledge of many aspects of health and public services, derived from over 15 years of working in and with many aspects of healthcare delivery. She was the

General Administrator of the Royal College of General Practitioners from 1984–94, and was President of the Association of Managers in General Practice (AMGP) from 1990–94. She chaired Newcastle City Health NHS Trust from its inception in 1993 to 1999. Currently she is appointed a lay member of the General Dental Council and an Arbitrator for the Arbitration and Conciliation Advisory Service.

In recent years she has concentrated on her work as a professional practice consultant in primary care working with her partner, Hilary Haman. She writes extensively on organisational and development issues within primary care, including seminal texts on audit and quality management, and writes regularly for the professional press. She was made an Honorary Fellow of the RCGP in 1995 and a Fellow of the AMGP in the same year. She is a Member of the Institute of Healthcare Management. She lives with her husband, Donald, in Northumberland and has three stepchildren and five grandchildren.

Di Jelley has been a general practitioner for 11 years in the North East of England, having taken a degree in sociology and worked in Mozambique as a teacher before going on to medical school. She combines general practice with both clinical and educational research, and is employed as an educational research fellow by the Northern Deanery Postgraduate Institute. She is currently completing a doctoral dissertation on the topic of peer appraisal. She worked for 10 years as an undergraduate teacher at Newcastle Medical School in the Department of Primary Healthcare until 1999, and she is a general practice trainer. She has also organised the Royal College of General Practitioners' Portuguese Exchange Programme for the last 10 years, and won the 1998 Marshall Marinker prize for excellence in general practice. She lives in Tynemouth with her husband and four children, and divides her personal time between family, friends and supporting Newcastle United.

Acknowledgements

This book is the product of our joint experience facilitating development within general practice, addressing areas such as team building, management and quality issues. We would all like to thank the many people in primary care who have participated in such occasions, and who have provided the impetus and foundation for this handbook.

The handbook represents our views but we are very grateful to Dr Colin Hunter and Brenda Sawyer for their invaluable suggestions and constructive comments. Professor Janet Gale Grant gave generous support in making the handbook easy to read and use. Sally Irvine would like to thank Professor Pauline McAvoy for working with her on the principles behind peer appraisal, and Di Jelley would like to thank all her colleagues at Collingwood Surgery for their support and encouragement, and particularly her partners for their willing engagement in various prototype peer appraisal sessions. Her thanks also to Professor Madeline Atkins for ongoing academic support, and to Professor Tim van Zwanenberg for many years of inspiration and vision.

We would all like to acknowledge the debt to our families in terms of time, intellectual challenge and encouragement, as well as tolerance and patience. This book is dedicated to them.

What this handbook aims to do

Peer appraisal is an effective way of helping people analyse and reflect on their work with those colleagues who can give insights into performance, attitudes and behaviours. Many general practitioners may wonder why they should consider setting up peer appraisal systems when they are already overburdened with clinical and administrative tasks. The answer is simple – appraisal can be an immensely useful and stimulating process for individuals and for the practice. It has the potential to change both the appraisee's and the organisation's performance, and to improve the quality of care delivered to patients. Appraisal has a key role in raising morale through feedback to colleagues that they are doing a very difficult job well, not just when they are doing less well. Peer appraisal will also provide a sound basis to prepare doctors for both external appraisal and revalidation.

General practitioners who responded to a recent study of peer appraisal in the North East of England identified a number of benefits that they felt had resulted from setting up peer appraisal systems. Some of them included the following:

- allowed us to know if our current practice was satisfactory and up to date
- provided a good starting point for the production of personal and practice development plans
- allowed us to share good practice and give each other support
- provided an important forum for reflection and feedback

- allowed us to identify strengths and weaknesses

- provided an opportunity to define our education and training needs

- improved confidence, morale and satisfaction of the doctors

- provided a safe environment to discuss difficult and complex issues

- improved teamwork and relationships in the partnership.

Our aim in this handbook is to provide a comprehensible and accessible framework for appraisal that readers can adapt to fit their individual needs. It is written to help any general practitioner, both working in partnership and single-handed, to become familiar and confident with appraisal. Non-principals such as: salaried assistants//locums// retainers//dental practitioners//and non-doctors including: practice managers, nurses, professions complementary to medicine and NHS managers will also find it useful as they meet the demands of clinical governance and revalidation.

Books and articles mentioned in the text are fully referenced on pp. 119–25.

The 10-step approach

Appraisal systems vary, but all successful schemes are likely to have addressed the following issues.

1   Purpose – what are the objectives of introducing a peer appraisal system?

2   Scope – what will be the content and range?

3   Collecting the information – how will the information needed for the appraisal be collected and collated?

4   Choosing the appraiser – who will carry out the appraisals?

5   Confidentiality – how is it related to the content and outcome of the appraisal system?

6   Administering the scheme – when, where and how often will the appraisal be carried out?

7   Training – what are the training needs of appraisers and appraisees?

8   The appraisal interview – how will it be conducted?

9   Recording the outcome – what records will be kept and by whom?

10 Reviewing the process – how will the system be reviewed and revised?

The 10 steps we describe in this handbook and as set out here will help you answer these questions.

10 steps in peer appraisal

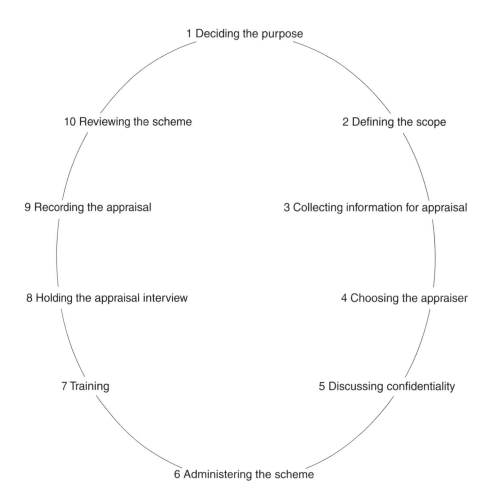

1 Deciding the purpose

10 Reviewing the scheme

2 Defining the scope

9 Recording the appraisal

3 Collecting information for appraisal

8 Holding the appraisal interview

4 Choosing the appraiser

7 Training

5 Discussing confidentiality

6 Administering the scheme

Why peer appraisal?

Appraisal and assessment:
are they different?

It is important at the outset to be clear about the terms we use in this book. Appraisal and assessment are frequently used almost interchangeably, but although they are linked concepts there are also significant differences between them and this handbook is clear about the differentiation. Generally, appraisal is considered to be a formative process of review, whereas assessment is a summative one. In simple terms, the former describes a developmental approach to performance based, non-judgemental but challenging and repeated review, whereas the latter has a significant element of 'pass/fail' in its approach, relying mostly on testing knowledge and skill against clear and explicit markers. Appraisal is usually a repeated process based on an ongoing working relationship between the appraisee and appraiser, and is therefore best conducted by a 'peer' or colleague, or someone directly managing the appraisee. Assessment is not based on any such relationship and can therefore be done by external assessors.

Why appraisal is so important

Appraisal has been a significant tool in the motivational approaches to management for many years across the commercial, industrial and public sectors. Indeed many corporate organisations, such as the Civil

Service, the British Broadcasting Corporation and local government institutions, have employed it successfully, largely in non-professional areas. It has also been introduced into education as part of a process of reviewing performance, identifying training needs and encouraging personal development. Appraisal has recently become an integral part of the institutional framework of the healthcare system in this country.

The current primary healthcare agenda emphasises quality standards and performance review via external appraisal as key mechanisms to improve the quality of healthcare delivery. Management-led clinical governance and professional-led revalidation have both cited appraisal as a principal means for promoting and monitoring the safe and effective performance of doctors and primary healthcare teams. Moreover, setting up a robust peer appraisal system for doctors prepares the ground for the extension of development plans to the whole team.

Doctors and dentists in training should be having their skills, achievements and further educational needs discussed with senior colleagues on a regular basis. Nurses and other professions allied to medicine have regular appraisal built into their training programmes. Many practice managers in primary care, with support if not involvement of clinical partners, have introduced staff appraisals into their teams. Often they have drawn on management expertise from outside the health service, or used models from schemes such as *Investors in People*.

All these appraisal systems, and those used in industry and education, have been designed generally to meet the needs of the hierarchical structure that is found in managed organisations. General practice partnerships have a more egalitarian structure, which require the basic principles of appraisal to be adapted appropriately to meet the different needs of a system based on peer review.

The General Medical Council (GMC), the Royal College of General Practitioners (RCGP) and the Department of Health (DoH) have all addressed this issue in recent years. For the GMC, a basic element of revalidation will be regular formative appraisal. Such appraisals are defined in its consultation document on revalidation as:

'regular opportunities in which a doctor is able, in a supportive environment, to identify and to discuss concerns with a colleague and to put things right.'

These proposals for revalidation assume that every general practitioner will be appraised annually in an individual interview carried out by a general practitioner colleague from outside the practice, who has been specially trained. During such an external appraisal interview the appraisee's educational activity, clinical performance and professional development will be discussed, supported by documentation from practice activity audits and feedback from colleagues and patients. Importantly, it is clear that any concerns about actual fitness to practise will be addressed by the appraiser outside the context of the appraisal interview.

The RCGP describes appraisal as a rigorous discussion between the general practitioner and an external peer, reviewing the strengths and weaknesses of the doctor's current performance. The outcome should be the agreement of a development plan, which will consolidate good practice and address areas of weakness.

The DoH, in *Supporting Doctors, Protecting Patients*, also emphasised the important role of appraisal. This document states that:

'Appraisal is a positive process to give someone feedback on their performance, to chart their continuing progress and to identify development needs.'

Additionally, in a recent interview the Chief Medical Officer (England) (CMO) confirmed that appraisal is a positive supportive process, a way of helping doctors develop and improve their performance and careers.

All these organisations describe a model of appraisal for general practice based on an individual interview with an *external* appraiser. There is no evidence available to confirm that this is the best way to set up appraisal in general practice. On the contrary, there is a strong argument that appraisal carried out within the practice and based on feedback from primary healthcare team colleagues and patients is more likely to lead to constructive and informative review. It is, moreover, an integral part of clinical governance and will provide a firm foundation for professional revalidation.

This handbook suggests that it is the process of peer appraisal within practices that has the greatest potential both to deliver the developmental aims of formative appraisal, and to encourage reflective practice within the primary care team. A robust team-based in-house appraisal system will be a central element in this process. We are clear that a rigorous, well-planned system of peer appraisal based on the sort of approach we describe in this handbook will be the best means for you and your partners to prepare for both external annual appraisal and revalidation.

We have already reflected the views of some general practitioners on the benefits of appraisal for them. Haman and Irvine (HIA) have summarised the benefits for individual practices and practitioners further:

- to identify and correct factors that may impair performance

- to develop a more collaborative style of managing the practice

- to identify training and personal development needs; essential for PDPs

- to reinforce effective behaviour and performance

- to assess how individuals can best contribute to achieving the aims of the practice

- to identify where there is duplication of effort

- to pinpoint time spent on tasks which have become obsolete

- to identify and avoid important gaps in knowledge and skills

- to create challenges for those who wish to undertake new activities

- to identify the educational needs of the practice.

The setting of a 'no blame' culture

Appraisal, even in the form demanded by the national institutions quoted, needs to be robust and will be highly dependent on the capacity and confidence of the appraisee to self-appraise. *An Organisation with a Memory* states that 'there is little culture of individual self-appraisal [in the NHS]' and that 'all those responsible for the initial and continuing training of doctors, nurses and other clinicians should address the developments of an approach to frank self-appraisal'. This represents a recognition by government (if not society) that in order to have successful appraisal it is crucial to set it in a blame-free culture. Such a culture will create an environment which is open, honest, safe, supportive and confidential, and yet rigorous and challenging – exactly the conditions needed for effective appraisal. If this culture is achieved then the organisation itself is more likely to be aware of and address poor performance and failures. Self-appraisal leads to self-improvement. Where there is a culture of blame, the opposite will occur; the knowledge and the information needed to address concerns of performance and quality will be driven underground.

How to use this handbook

Our aim in this handbook is to help you and your practice set up supportive peer appraisal that provides first, insight into personal motivations for the individual (through encouraging self-appraisal), and second, a focus on team expectations and development priorities for you and your practice. It is an opportunity to identify weaknesses but, equally important, to give positive feedback to peers, encouraging and rewarding good performance.

We are conscious that we also need to address legitimate and natural concerns about peer appraisal in those who have little or negative experience of its use. In the study in Northern England mentioned earlier, general practitioners reflected some of these fears:

- the threats and fears of receiving negative feedback

- the lack of time and resources to carry out appraisals effectively

- the difficulties of getting everyone to take part

- the lack of skills of the potential appraiser

- the destructive impact of badly conducted appraisals

- the difficulties of finding an appropriate appraiser.

To meet these fears and to deliver the identified and agreed benefits, this handbook describes how you can achieve a peer appraisal system that is a developmental rather than a punitive or judgemental experience. We have included a section on how to give constructive feedback (in Step 7) which we hope, if followed, will take away some of the fears and threats associated with the appraisal process. It is also important that you are clear at the outset that you cannot do it all at once, but should see the development of the system as an ongoing and progressive process, to be tackled systematically but paced to reflect your local circumstances. The key is to work through the tools provided – they are listed in Box 1 for reference.

You may wish to adapt the Toolsheets for your specific needs. However, if you want further sets of the Toolsheets as printed in this book, please contact HIA (*see* p. 125 for contact details).

How to use this handbook 9

Box 1 The steps and tools

Step		Tool	Page
1 Deciding the purpose	1	Clarifying the reasons for introducing a peer appraisal scheme	15
2 Defining the scope	2.1	Choosing appraisal priorities	21
	2.2	The scope of the practice peer appraisal scheme	22
3 Collecting information for appraisal	3.1	Partners' video feedback form	27
	3.2	Patient's consent to videoing consultation	29
	3.3	Identifying Doctors' Educational Needs (DENs) using a log diary	31
	3.4	Significant event discussion record	33
	3.5	Patient feedback	35
	3.6	Team feedback questionnaire	37
	3.7	Staff assessment rating form	38
	3.8	Learning diary	42
	3.9	Self-assessment: GP health questionnaire	44
	3.10	Collating information for the appraisal	47
4 Choosing the appraiser	4	Appraisal by whom? An agenda for group discussion	55
5 Discussing confidentiality	5	Confidentiality discussion checklist	62
6 Administering the scheme	6	Administrative essentials	69
7 Training	7	Identifying appraisal skills	74
8 Holding the appraisal interview	8.1	Sample pre-appraisal form for the appraisee	86
	8.2	Sample pre-appraisal form for the appraiser(s)	89
	8.3	Ideas for opening appraisal interviews	92
	8.4	Sample appraisal interview agenda	95
	8.5	Raising sensitive issues	96
	8.6	Appraisal action plan	98
9 Recording the appraisal	9	A personal development plan	106
10 Reviewing the scheme	10.1	The short-term review	111
	10.2	The longer-term review	112

It is crucial that all partners and as many of the primary care team as possible are involved in the development of the appraisal process for it to be truly effective and rigorous. Box 2 shows the possible time-scales for completing the 10 steps, with suggestions as to who should be involved at which points.

Box 2   Actions and timeframe for the 10-step approach

Action	Who is involved?	Time taken (hours)	Comments
Agree to develop peer appraisal system	All partners/all doctors	Unlimited	Essential first stage – there must be commitment
Meet to discuss and record practice decisions on Steps 1–6	All partners/ doctors/practice manager	1–2 hours	May need more than one meeting
Identify training needs of scheme and plan training if necessary	All partners/ doctors/ administrator	1–3 hours	
Carry out training	All partners/ doctors	4–8 hours	Depending on availability of courses
Carry out interviews – individual or group	All partners	1 hour per interview	
Collate training outcomes of individual interviews	All partners/ administrator	1 hour	
Review scheme	All partners/ doctors/ administrator	1 hour	

You are now ready to start the planning of a peer appraisal system that will suit your partnership and its current stage of development. Most of the tools in this handbook can also be readily adapted for use by other members of the primary care team. When the appraisal system has been set up, each individual should be able to produce a personal development plan based on the outcomes of the appraisal meeting. If the other members of the primary care team are also involved these can then be linked to produce a practice development plan.

Do be aware, however, that peer appraisal is not an appropriate tool for addressing longstanding partnership disputes, nor is it likely to be viable in a seriously dysfunctional partnership. In these latter circumstances external facilitation and support may be useful, as almost certainly outside help will be needed.

Step 1 Purpose of the scheme

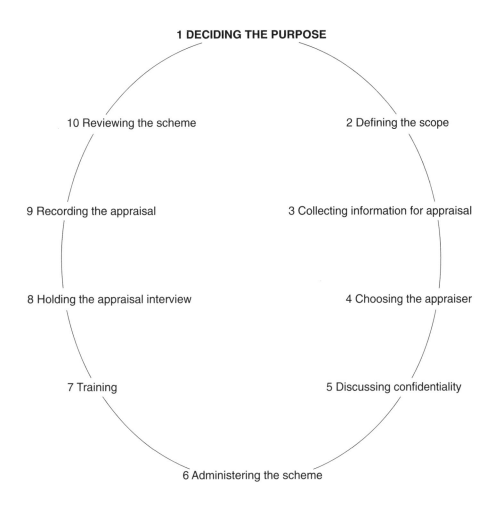

1 DECIDING THE PURPOSE

10 Reviewing the scheme

2 Defining the scope

9 Recording the appraisal

3 Collecting information for appraisal

8 Holding the appraisal interview

4 Choosing the appraiser

7 Training

5 Discussing confidentiality

6 Administering the scheme

Step 1 | Deciding the purpose: objectives of a peer appraisal scheme

For you and your colleagues to feel committed to any activity, you need to understand and agree the reasons why it is being carried out. This is particularly true for a process such as peer appraisal. Generally speaking it will be outside the personal experience of most general practitioners, and may seem threatening and difficult to carry out. This makes it all the more critically important for you and your colleagues in the practice to discuss together at the outset why you want to set up such a system and what you all hope to gain from doing so. The discussion of the benefits and outcomes of peer appraisal on pp. 1–4 may be helpful background for these discussions.

Practices vary a great deal in terms of workload, demography, resources, organisational systems, computerisation etc., and therefore the shape and aims of peer appraisal schemes will vary enormously. It is thus very important to define a system whose shape and scope will suit the needs of your practice.

Tool 1 is a framework to help you and your practice establish an agenda for a practice meeting where you can clarify your ideas in this area.

Tool 1   Clarifying the reasons for introducing a peer appraisal scheme

1   The main reasons for introducing the scheme are:

2   The main purpose of the scheme is:

3   The benefits to the appraisees will be:

4   The benefits to the practice will be:

5   Any other specific issues within the partnership or the practice that could be addressed through the introduction of peer appraisal:

Step 2 Defining the scope of the scheme: what to appraise

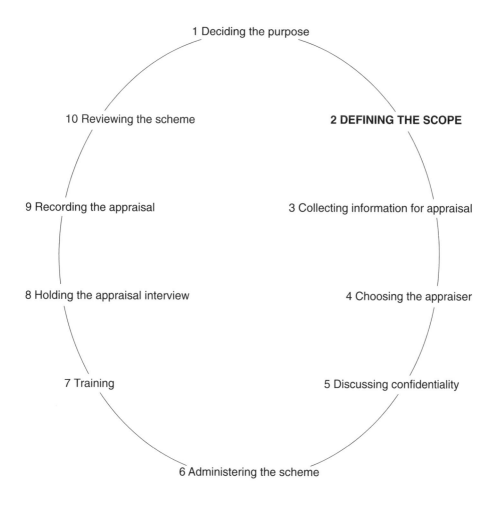

1 Deciding the purpose

10 Reviewing the scheme

2 DEFINING THE SCOPE

9 Recording the appraisal

3 Collecting information for appraisal

8 Holding the appraisal interview

4 Choosing the appraiser

7 Training

5 Discussing confidentiality

6 Administering the scheme

Step 2 Defining the scope: what to appraise

Having agreed the purpose, the next step in designing a scheme is to clarify what areas are to be covered. The range of clinical and non-clinical issues that make up each general practitioner's workload is vast, and obviously each appraisal meeting can only cover a few areas. It is important that everybody is clear what the focus is to be for the first peer appraisal meeting, so that interview processes can be consistent and comprehensive.

As we have discussed (see p. 4) there is a clear link between appraisal and revalidation. It is therefore sensible when deciding on the scope of your scheme to reflect the broad framework to be covered by revalidation. Fortunately there is clear guidance here. The GMC has laid down the areas of good practice in *Good Medical Practice*, and it is these that will form the criteria for revalidation. The RCGP has tailored those areas for general practice in its document *Good Medical Practice for General Practitioners*. It is the latter that we are using here. You and your colleagues can review the full range together. Box 3 provides a checklist, derived from *Good Medical Practice for General Practitioners*, which you may find helpful when having this discussion.

Box 3   Scope for appraisal

Main sections	*Sub-sections*
1 Good clinical care	1 Clinical care 2 Keeping records/informing colleagues 3 Access and availability 4 Emergency treatment 5 Out-of-hours care 6 Effective use of resources
2 Maintaining good practice	7 Keeping up to date – maintaining your performance
3 Good relationships with patients	8 Providing information to patients 9 Professional relationships with patients 10 Avoiding discrimination and prejudice 11 If things go wrong
4 Working with colleagues	12 Working with colleagues/ working in teams 13 Referring patients 14 Responsibilities of specialists 15 Accepting posts
5 Teaching and training	16 Teaching and training
6 Probity	17 Research 18 Abusing your professional position 19 Financial dealings · 20 Providing references
7 Performance of other doctors	21 Protecting patients when a doctor's health, conduct or performance puts them at risk

Within these broad categories, you will want to decide for your-selves which of the sub-categories under these headings are of most significance for your practice at this time. Tool 2.1 is a form for each partner to use to decide and prioritise which are most important for him/her, and which are most important for the practice – they are not always the same thing. Tool 2.2 provides a proforma to pull together the results of the group discussion.

Tool 2.1 Choosing appraisal priorities

Using the areas set out in *Good Medical Practice for General Practitioners*, the following are my priorities for me and for the practice:

For me	For the practice	High/medium or low (H, M, L) priority

Tool 2.2   The scope of the practice peer appraisal scheme

Main sections		Sub-sections	High/medium or low (H, M, L) priority
1	Good clinical care	1 Clinical care 2 Keeping records/informing colleagues 3 Access and availability 4 Emergency treatment 5 Out-of-hours care 6 Effective use of resources	
2	Maintaining good practice	7 Keeping up to date – maintaining your performance	
3	Good relationships with patients	8 Providing information to patients 9 Professional relationships with patients 10 Avoiding discrimination and prejudice 11 If things go wrong	
4	Working with colleagues	12 Working with colleagues/working in teams 13 Referring patients 14 Responsibilities of specialists 15 Accepting posts	
5	Teaching and training	16 Teaching and training	
6	Probity	17 Research 18 Abusing your professional position 19 Financial dealings 20 Providing references	
7	Performance of other doctors	21 Protecting patients when a doctor's health, conduct or performance puts them at risk	
	Any additional areas		

Step 3 Collecting information for appraisal

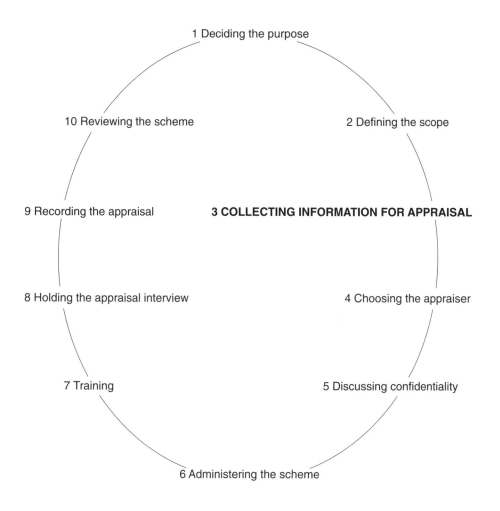

1 Deciding the purpose

10 Reviewing the scheme

2 Defining the scope

9 Recording the appraisal

3 COLLECTING INFORMATION FOR APPRAISAL

8 Holding the appraisal interview

4 Choosing the appraiser

7 Training

5 Discussing confidentiality

6 Administering the scheme

Step 3 Collecting information for appraisal

As we have seen in the steps taken so far, peer appraisal can address both clinical and non-clinical aspects of your work. In Step 2 you will have spent some time considering what will be the main focus of each partner's appraisal within the broad framework of *Good Medical Practice for General Practitioners*. Your appraisal interview will provide an opportunity to share your and others' feedback on your performance in the areas you have chosen to review, as well as any more general key issues. Making the most of this time often requires information to be collected by you and your partners, which can support the comments made at the appraisal meeting. Considering what data might be helpful and how it might be collected is the next step.

Box 4 summarises a wide range of methods for collecting information in relation to each section of *Good Medical Practice for General Practitioners*. Some are less relevant to the early stages of introducing peer appraisal and they are fully referenced in the Appendix for you and your partners to look at when the need arises. We discuss here the methods that are the most common and probably the most useful to you in developing appraisal systems. They are marked in bold in the box and in the following pages are described in turn. Tools 8.1–8.6 as described in Step 8 are useful in implementing them.

Box 4   Collecting information for peer appraisal

Main sections	Sub-sections	Methods of collecting information
1 Good clinical care	Clinical care Keeping records/ informing colleagues Access and availability Emergency treatment Out-of-hours care Effective use of resources	**Video** ● Clinical audit ● Multiple choice questions (MCQs) ● Rating scales ● **Log diaries/significant event auditing**/clinical meetings; Case analysis; **Patient feedback** ● Telephone access and appointment audits ● Case analysis ● **Significant event audits** ● MCQs skill reviews ● **Patient feedback**; Case analysis; Clinical and admin audit ● PACT data; Pharmacist feedback; PCT-level PACT review
2 Maintaining good practice	Keeping up to date – maintaining your performance	● MCQs ● **Learning diaries** ● Review of external educational events ● Clinical meetings in practice
3 Good relationships with patients	Providing information to patients Professional relationships with patients Avoiding discrimination and predjudice If things go wrong	● **Formal and informal feedback from patients via surgery, receptionists, clinical team and colleagues** ● Regular review of complaints ● **Significant event analysis**
4 Working with colleagues	Working with colleagues/ working in teams Referring patients Responsibilities of specialists Accepting posts	● **Formal feedback from colleagues via questionnaires** ● **360° appraisal** ● Team meetings ● Review of referrals ● Discussions/meetings with secondary care colleagues
5 Teaching and training	Teaching and training	● Review + updating of teaching and training responsibilities and skills ● **Patient feedback on trainees + impact of teaching on patient care**
6 Probity	Research Abusing your professional position Financial dealings Providing references	● Review of impact of research on practice and patients ● Clinical audit re implementation of research findings
7 Performance of other doctors	Protecting patients when a doctor's health, conduct or performance puts them at risk	● **Regular review of stress in self and others**

Note: methods in bold type are discussed in more detail in this chapter.

Video consultations

In the education sector, appraisal in teaching is based on information gained by direct observation of classroom practice. In medicine there is a wealth of evidence to support the use of video in improving consultation skills and encouraging reflection on what happened in the consultation and why. Video taping of consultations is part of a registrar's day-to-day life, but there are many general practice principals who have never seen themselves (let alone their partners) consult. The use of video can be threatening in such circumstances.

If you have not used video before, you might start by viewing tapes of your consultations alone. You may then feel emboldened to view them with a trusted colleague. There are many methods of analysing consultation on video and as a starting point, Tool 3.1 is included here. It is based on partners watching each other's videos, using the MRCGP examination questions as a guide. There are some rules however. As with most situations, negative criticism without constructive suggestion is poorly received and unhelpful.

As confidence increases, it is very helpful to watch the whole tape through with colleagues and allow the doctor to define any key issues to address, using Tool 3.1 as a guide. Then rewind the tape and replay it, stopping it frequently to ask questions such as:

- what were you thinking at that moment?
- what else could you have said?
- what would have happened if you had said nothing then?
- what was the patient feeling at that time?

Tool 3.1 Partners' video feedback form

Criteria		Yes	No	Comments
1	Is the patient's contribution encouraged?	☐	☐	
2	Are cues picked up and addressed?	☐	☐	
3	Is the patient's social and psychological context explored, if appropriate?	☐	☐	
4	Is an appropriate examination carried out?	☐	☐	
5	Is an appropriate diagnosis made?	☐	☐	
6	Is the management plan appropriate?	☐	☐	
7	Is the diagnosis and management plan explained to the patient?	☐	☐	
8	Is the language used understandable to the patient?	☐	☐	
9	Are management options shared with the patient?	☐	☐	
10	Is the prescription issued appropriate?	☐	☐	

© 2001 Haman, Irvine and Jelley

Patient consent

The issue of patient consent needs to be well thought out and prepared in advance. For instance, it is important to have a protocol
whereby patients are told when they book an appointment that the
surgery will be videoed. This will give them time to think about
whether they object or not. If they do not, then signed permission for
video taping the consultation must be obtained from every patient.
Tool 3.2 gives a sample consent form. It needs to be handed to the
patient when they arrive at reception. It also needs to be signed again
after the consultation and handed back to you or the reception desk.
Videotapes of consultations should be kept securely with the consent
forms and wiped clean after they have been viewed and discussed.

Tool 3.2   Patient's consent to videoing consultation

Patient's name: ....   Date: ....

Consent to video recording for doctor assessment purposes

We are hoping to make video recordings of some of the consultations between patients and Dr .... You are seeing Dr .... today.

The videos are part of a regular appraisal procedure we have in this practice which helps to make sure that all of the doctors who treat you are fully up to date.

The video is **only** of you and the doctor talking together. No intimate examination will be done in front of the camera. All video recordings are carried out according to guidance issued by the General Medical Council.

The video will be seen only by doctors and the tape will then be erased (usually within four weeks of recording, and in any event within one year). The tape will be stored in a locked cabinet and has the same level of confidentiality and security as your medical record. Dr .... is personally responsible for the security and confidentiality of the video recording. In the unlikely event that the tape has to leave the practice premises, it will normally be in the possession of the doctor. If it is necessary to send it to another doctor or doctors as part of the appraisal process, it will be sent by registered post or personal messenger. If you want to see the tape recording, please ask the receptionist.

You do not have to agree to your consultation with the doctor being recorded. If you want the camera turned off, please tell Reception – this is not a problem and will not affect your consultation in any way. But if you do not mind your consultation being recorded, we are grateful to you. Giving doctors these sorts of opportunities to reflect on their performance with colleagues should lead to a better service for patients.

If you consent to this consultation being recorded, please sign below. Thank you very much for your help.

Signed: ....   Date: ....

After you have finished seeing the doctor, please sign below to confirm that you are still happy to have the recording used.

Signed: ....   Date: ....

Log diaries

Log diaries are a simple but powerful way of defining educational needs in both clinical and non-clinical areas. It is a technique used by GP registrars to record questions and teaching points associated with specific patients they have seen. Richard Eve has developed a slightly more elaborate system for use by established general practitioners. He uses a diary format and encourages general practitioners to record information about any consultation in which they feel on reflection the patient had an 'unmet need' (PUN). He suggests the doctor then tries to define the educational needs (DEN), which when addressed would meet the patient's unmet need. More details of how to obtain copies of log books with worked examples are given on p. 123.

Educational needs defined using log diaries are necessarily subjective but can provide useful material to discuss, particularly at a group-based peer appraisal meeting. Such diaries can often throw up a plethora of needs. Getting feedback from colleagues about their needs defined in this way can help provide some consensus for establishing priorities.

A sample diary sheet is attached as Tool 3.3.

Tool 3.3   Identifying Doctors' Educational Needs (DENs) using a log diary

For any consultation fill in this sheet. It is best to do so when you have a few minutes to think and reflect, especially if a consultation has been difficult or challenging. The sheet does not have to be completed for every patient contact.

Doctor: ....   Date: ....

Patient name or number	Presenting problem and challenges (Patient's Unmet Needs – PUNs)	Doctor's Educational Need (DEN). How could I have done it better?

© Richard Eve

Significant event auditing

This is an extremely useful tool, which can involve the whole team in discussing a wide range of clinical problems – often those with adverse outcomes. The idea is to analyse and dissect all the activities that led up to the significant event concerned, and from that analysis share views on what could have been done differently. The basic questions asked are:

- what went well?
- what went badly?
- how could I/we improve?

Common examples of suitable events for this sort of treatment might include:

- the death of a young adult from ischaemic heart disease
- pregnancy in a young teenager
- late diagnosis of inoperable cancer
- suicide in a patient well-known to the practice
- a diabetic patient admitted in keto-acidosis.

The aim of subjecting them to analysis is to learn from what happened and, if appropriate, to identify any training needs. A common format is for a summary of the case to be presented to the team and for the management decisions taken at each stage to be reviewed in a 'no blame' culture. This process is described in more depth by Rughani (2000) and in an article by Robinson, Story and Spencer. Lessons learned and educational needs defined are agreed, recorded and circulated after the meetings. These may be reviewed at the peer appraisal meeting. These events, and there are many other examples, occur in every practice.

Tool 3.4 can be used to record a summary of significant event discussions.

Tool 3.4   Significant event discussion record

Significant event meeting on: ....

Brief summary of event:

Main issues arising from the discussion:
1

2

3

Positive feedback:
1

2

3

Areas of concern:
1

2

3

Suggestions for action   _Person responsible_

1
2
3
4

Patients' views

This is probably the hardest set of data to obtain, partly because of the time involved in collecting it, and partly because patient satisfaction surveys often tell us little of specific value. Most patients are satisfied most of the time – to move beyond this limited view it is probably necessary to ask patients face-to-face for specific examples of when the doctor functioned very well and less well.

Receptionists are often a rich source of patient feedback about specific doctors, but it is often difficult to formalise this to enable it to be used in an appraisal interview. Keeping an anonymous patients' comments book, including positive and negative remarks, can sometimes be revealing and provoke discussion.

Patients' complaints are an important source of feedback for the practice as a whole and for the individual doctor. They provide important material that can be discussed at an appraisal meeting but, clearly, any critical issues will need to be addressed as they arise. A recent publication by Ruth Chambers, explores these issues in much greater depth and gives explicit guidance on involving patients in providing feedback to practices. The National Clinical Audit Centre at the Department of General Practice in Leicester has developed an easy to administer consultation satisfaction questionnaire – for details *see* p. 123.

We include Tool 3.5 as an additional aid based on patient feedback for doctors to reflect on before their appraisal meeting.

Tool 3.5 Patient feedback

Think back over the last three months and use this sheet to record briefly one recent positive and one recent negative comment from a patient, and the lessons learned from each.

	Comment	Lessons learned
Positive		
Negative		

Team feedback

Your effectiveness as a general practitioner will depend in large part on your functioning within the primary care team. Obtaining direct feedback from your employees (the administrative team and the practice nursing team) is often resisted by both sides. However, it may be possible to persuade your team to complete feedback questionnaires or to give verbal feedback to your practice manager. If so, some important issues may emerge which can be discussed at the appraisal meeting. It is sometimes easier to receive such feedback in the context of a group appraisal meeting if the lead appraiser ensures everyone is hearing some praise and some criticism.

Tools 3.6 and 3.7 are examples of feedback questionnaires. The first, Tool 3.6, covers the key areas of good medical practice that could be useful for members of the primary care team to provide feedback to individual doctors. Tool 3.7 is an adaptation of a staff trainee assessment form devised by North Northumberland Trainer Group. They are both included because in some practices staff will only give feedback on the doctors (their employers) if anonymity is guaranteed using a 'tick box' format.

Tool 3.6 Team feedback questionnaire

Feedback questionnaire for Dr .... Date ....

Area	What are the Dr's strengths in this area?	Where could there be improvement?
1 Good clinical care		
2 Keeping up to date		
3 Good relations with patients		
4 Working with colleagues		
5 Teaching and training		

Tool 3.7 Staff assessment rating form

This form contains a number of statements about the doctor named below. Please tick your perceived agreement/disagreement with the statements, and return the completed form in the envelope provided. The answers will be kept entirely confidential, so please be honest in your responses.

Doctor .... Date ....

	Strongly agree 5	Agree 4	Neutral 3	Disagree 2	Disagree strongly 1
The doctor is always polite and courteous	☐	☐	☐	☐	☐
He/she always conducts him/herself in a professional manner	☐	☐	☐	☐	☐
He/she is happy to accept any extra duties	☐	☐	☐	☐	☐
He/she is always punctual and invariably keeps to time schedules	☐	☐	☐	☐	☐
He/she appears keen to seek my help and advice	☐	☐	☐	☐	☐
He/she is able to accept criticism	☐	☐	☐	☐	☐
He/she appreciates my role and skills	☐	☐	☐	☐	☐
He/she works in a well-organised manner	☐	☐	☐	☐	☐
He/she appears to be well-liked by patients	☐	☐	☐	☐	☐
He/she is very easy to get on with and fits well in the team	☐	☐	☐	☐	☐

There are, however, some concerns with the use of such forms. The appraiser obtains the feedback but the appraisee needs to know who is giving the feedback and what areas are under discussion. The appraiser has an important screening role in passing on this feedback, without undermining the relationships within the team. The success of this is highly dependent on the proper resolution of the issues of trust and confidentiality which we discuss in Step 5. Suffice to note here that you may need to give guarantees of anonymity when first using such a questionnaire, until everyone has confidence in certain aspects of the appraiser's use of the feedback.

You and your partners need to encourage the team to focus on areas of a doctor's performance that can be improved and put right. These would include such things as losing notes or issues of poor communication, rather than personal aspects such as child care commitments and the need to leave at a fixed time, which are difficult to change. The golden rule is only to deal with and challenge what people do, not what they are. Learning how to deliver appropriate feedback is discussed at greater length in Step 7.

360° feedback

A particular method of eliciting team feedback is called 360° Appraisal. 360° feedback is the process of collecting perceptions from a number of respondents such as:

- your line manager (or managers)

- at least three people for whose work you are directly responsible

- at least three of your peers/colleagues

- possibly some patients and other colleagues who know you well.

All these perceptions, from different angles, are then compared and contrasted with your perceptions of yourself, so that you can discover your strengths and weaknesses.

You can make 360° feedback more selective. For instance, you can limit it to those who report directly to you or, alternatively, you may prefer to concentrate on the perceptions of particular colleagues. Obviously, the wider the collection the more effective the process, but equally the design of the questionnaire is all important.

This model has been adapted for use in some general practices. Uni-disciplinary groups of nurses, reception staff and doctors all design their own feedback questionnaires. Each individual gives their questionnaire to three people, one from each group, whom they select. A fourth person receives each person's three questionnaires, collates and, if necessary, moderates the feedback, and then discusses it with each person individually. *Insight*, a computerised tool to elicit feedback in this way is available from Edgecumbe Consulting (*see* p. 124 for full details on how to obtain this tool).

360° feedback is widely used in large organisations but probably has a limited role in the small but complex structure of general practice partnerships, not least because it can generate hurtful and unsubstantiated comment to which the recipient cannot adequately respond.

Learning diaries

The process of identifying and monitoring learning needs is greatly facilitated by keeping a paper- or computer-based learning diary, which can be completed periodically in the time between appraisals. Tool 3.8 is an example of a simple diary format that can easily be put on to the computer. Notes can be made from issues that arise in the consultation, during formal or informal practice meetings, or from reading journals, watching television, attending educational courses etc.

Tool 3.8 Learning diary

Learning situation	Learning outcomes	Actions planned

Review of stress in yourself

Working as a general practitioner is without doubt a stressful job. This is not just in terms of the clinical challenge but also because of the emotional impact of much of the work. In addition, there is now a high volume of administrative tasks both for accountability and validation of professional judgement facing the primary care team. The importance of finding an opportunity for reflection on your own health is highlighted in Section 7 of the GMC's *Good Medical Practice*, and the appraisal meeting provides a chance to do this.

Delivering high-quality clinical care not only requires up to date knowledge and skills but also needs you to be physically and mentally fit enough to consult with patients, work in a team and have a fulfilling life outside work. Some recent useful publications to help doctors in this area are listed on p. 123. Tool 3.9 is a self-assessment questionnaire designed by Dr Barbara Scott, a general practitioner in Cleveland, which will help you identify any areas for concern in your personal functioning which you might want to bring to the appraisal meeting.

Tool 3.9   Self-assessment: GP health questionnaire

The purpose of this questionnaire is to encourage you to reflect on your own general health and well-being so that your performance and enjoyment of your work is not compromised in any way. *If you answer No to any question, consider doing something about it or seek help.*

General

		Yes	No
Are you up-to-date with:	Tetanus vaccinations?	☐	☐
	Hepatitis B immunity?	☐	☐
	Rubella immunity?	☐	☐
	Mammography?	☐	☐
	Cervical smears?	☐	☐
• Do you have a family history of significance?		☐	☐
• If so, have you taken steps to identify your own risks?		☐	☐
• Are you registered with a GP outside your practice?		☐	☐
• Are your family registered with a GP?		☐	☐
• Have you had less than two weeks off work due to illness in the last year?		☐	☐
• Have you made up-to-date financial provision for yourself and your family in the event of ill health?		☐	☐

Physical health

	Yes	No
• If appropriate have you had your BP/cholesterol checked in the past two years?	☐	☐
• If you have an existing medical condition, has it been reviewed appropriately?	☐	☐
• If you have any significant physical symptoms, have you discussed these with your GP?	☐	☐
• Do you manage to take regular exercise at least three times a week?	☐	☐
• Do you think you eat a varied diet with plenty of fruit and vegetables?	☐	☐

Stress and mental health

	Yes	No
• Do you work less than 55 hours per week?	☐	☐
• Count how many substantial life/work events have happened to you in the last year	....	

- Look at the human function curve – are you mostly in the healthy zone? ☐ ☐ ☐
- If you are feeling the effects of stress, have you considered seeking help?
- Do your answers indicate that your mental health is satisfactory? ☐ ☐

Substance abuse

- Is your alcohol intake within the recommended limits? ☐ ☐ ☐ ☐
- If you are a smoker, have you tried to stop?
- If you are using any addictive drug, have you considered getting help? ☐ ☐ ☐ ☐
- If you are using substantial self-medication for anything, have you considered modifying or ceasing the treatment?

Lifestyle

- Have you given some thought to the balance between work and play? ☐ ☐ ☐ ☐ ☐ ☐ ☐
- Do you take proper holidays?
- Do you have some hobbies or interests outside work?
- Do they take up at least one evening or afternoon a week? ☐ ☐ ☐ ☐ ☐ ☐ ☐
- Do you have enough energy left for these?
- Are you spending enough time with friends and family?
- Is your personal life fulfilling?

So what is your assessment of yourself?

- Is all well with you? ☐
- If you need to make some changes make a list of things to do ☐ ....

....

IF YOU CONSIDER YOUR PERFORMANCE AT WORK IS SUFFERING BECAUSE OF ILLNESS OR STRESS, NOW IS THE TIME TO SEEK HELP

Summary

When you have finished reading this section and the further information in the Appendix, use Box 3 (Scope for appraisal, p. 19) as the background for completing Tool 3.10 which enables you to summarise the methods and data you have decided to use. It is important to emphasise that you need to collect the relevant information before the appraisal meeting. Obviously, the videoed consultation or significant event or other activity will not be reviewed in depth at the appraisal meeting, but your (and your colleagues') feedback on the activity will be.

Tool 3.10   Collating information for the appraisal

1   Which broad areas do I wish to concentrate on during the appraisal interview?

2   What specific issues do I wish to raise?

3   Why do I wish to raise the above issues?

4   What information/data do I need in order to underline/exemplify this issue?

5   What methods can I use to collate this information?

Step 4 Choosing the appraiser

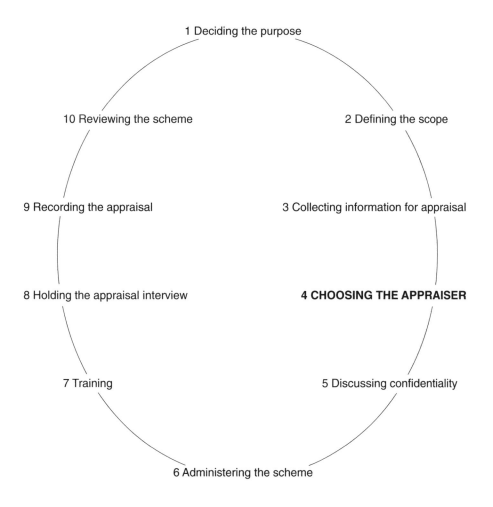

1 Deciding the purpose

10 Reviewing the scheme

2 Defining the scope

9 Recording the appraisal

3 Collecting information for appraisal

8 Holding the appraisal interview

4 CHOOSING THE APPRAISER

7 Training

5 Discussing confidentiality

6 Administering the scheme

Step 4 Choosing the appraiser: who should appraise?

Individual or group appraisal

This question of who does the appraisal is crucial. After deciding the purpose and the scope of the appraisal system to be used, together with the information and evidence to be used, the answer to this question will determine the shape of the scheme. It is a question that you need to discuss as a partnership group. This section will help to focus that discussion.

Peer appraisal, by definition, has to involve appraisal by another general practitioner who should:

- know the appraisee's work
- be able to handle sensitive issues
- be respected by the appraisee
- ideally be trained and confident in handling a peer appraisal interview.

This will generally lead to a member of the same practice working closely with the appraisee.

At this point in designing the scheme, the most important issue for you to address in your practice is whether your appraisal scheme should be based on:

- an appraisal interview conducted by one doctor colleague, or

- an interview conducted with each doctor in turn by a number of doctor colleagues in the form of a group interview, or

- in large practices the latter option may be further extended to allow the doctors to be divided into two or three smaller groups.

Each method has its advantages and disadvantages. These are outlined in Box 5 which provides a framework for all involved to work through to allow you all to discuss which method best suits your partnership at this time. It is important that this question is discussed with all the doctors and that the various options are explored, keeping in mind the broad objectives of the scheme that you defined in Tool 1 on p. 15.

Box 5 A comparison of individual and group-based appraisal

Criteria	Individual interviews	Group-based appraisal
1 Appraisal process	1 May be easier to discuss sensitive issues in a one-to-one interview	1 Shared knowledge between all parties of the key issues for each doctor
	2 Helps to avoid potentially destructive influence of pre-existing personality clashes on the appraisal process	2 May be easier for the practice to give constructive criticism, including staff feedback to doctors
	3 Individual may receive more time and focused attention	3 Easier to obtain feedback from all doctors to each partner and to share openly
	4 Easier to plan and run than a group interview	4 All doctors can experience both roles of appraiser and appraisee
	5 Does not need facilitation	
2 Outcomes	1 More focused individual appraisal time may produce more detailed and defined outcomes and aims	1 Easier to match personal development needs with those of the practice
	2 Easier to produce a personal development plan following an individual interview	2 Easier to produce a practice development plan, defining priorities for an individual's development needs
	3 Recording of discussion is easier	3 Shared discussion of strengths and weaknesses is a powerful way to develop team cohesion when handled sensitively

Issues for single-handed practice and non-principals

There are some particular issues relating to single-handed, very small, practices and non-principals in relation to appraisal which need to be dealt with here. They are set out in Box 6.

Box 6   Issues for single-handed practice and non-principals

These issues frequently relate to the belief that the absence of colleagues to participate in peer appraisal excludes such practices from undertaking peer appraisal. As a consequence we deal with the issue here, as we believe that all of the tools and activities described in this handbook could be used by a single-handed doctor, or doctors in a small practice, either through team appraisal or with peers across several practices.

Team appraisal
Primary care teams in small practices often have very close working relationships based on mutual respect. It is possible therefore for the team – doctors, nurses and non-clinical staff – to reflect together on how the practice is running. This reflection could include clinical and non-clinical performance and educational needs. This process can provide feedback to all members on areas such as communication within the team, relationships with colleagues and many aspects of practice administration. Many of the tools described in Step 3 could be useful here.

Peer appraisal
In terms of clinical competence, as single-handed practices, small practices and non-principals, you already work together in many areas – for instance, sharing your out-of-hours commitments, or in 'virtual practices' for non-principals. To set up peer appraisal between you would require resources to provide locum cover and protected time. If this is made available, then the same processes described in Steps 1 to 4 could be undertaken within a group of doctors from several small practices. The initial focus might be to share disease management or prescribing issues in specified areas, leading on to more challenging matters such as consultation skills, or significant event auditing. It might be worth approaching your local Postgraduate Institute of General Practice for support in making contact with other practices and providing some funding.

Alternatively, as a single-handed general practitioner without suitable local colleagues, you might seek out a mentor in another practice or the local primary care trust to enable you to gain the benefit of a colleague's views of your practice.

Whatever your situation, the tools in this book should be readily adaptable to allow you to discuss the setting up of an appraisal system with local colleagues.

So who will appraise?

When you have considered the merits of individual and group-based interviews, a decision will have to be made as to who will be the appraiser(s) in the practice. Will one person do all the individual interviews or lead the group meeting, or will these roles rotate? Working through Tool 4 as a group should enable you as a practice to reach a decision and have clear reasons.

Tool 4   Appraisal by whom? An agenda for group discussion

1   Is group or individual appraisal the best approach for our practice?

2   What are our reasons for choosing this model?

If we opt for individual interviews:

3   Who will be the appraiser?

4   Why were they chosen?

5   Will the appraisee choose his/her appraiser(s)?

6   If not, how will we identify the appraiser(s)?

7   Will the person(s) identified be the same for all the appraisals?

8   If so, who will appraise the appraiser?

If we opt for group-based interviews:

9   Who will lead the group meetings?

10   Will this responsibility rotate?

11   Will the practice manager be present?

Review
12   When and how will we review who should undertake the appraisal?

Step 5 Confidentiality

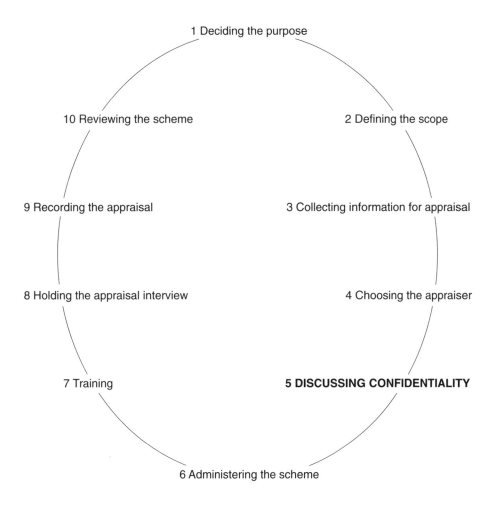

1 Deciding the purpose

10 Reviewing the scheme

2 Defining the scope

9 Recording the appraisal

3 Collecting information for appraisal

8 Holding the appraisal interview

4 Choosing the appraiser

7 Training

5 DISCUSSING CONFIDENTIALITY

6 Administering the scheme

Step 5 Discussing confidentiality

All doctors and other health professionals will be sensitive to issues of confidentiality in their professional lives, in relation to patient information, employees' data and practice matters. Appraisal raises some special and important dimensions to this subject. There is a danger, when a scheme is first designed, to assume that everything will be confidential. This is neither feasible nor efficacious. Confidentiality impinges on, and is central to, the various stages of the appraisal cycle, including the purpose of the scheme (Step 1), its range (Step 2) and what you hope to achieve from it. The type that you decided on in Step 4 (i.e. one-to-one interviews or group interviews) will determine the appropriate level and type of confidentiality.

Attitudes to confidentiality can be complex and it is important that you discuss it fully taking each of the steps in the appraisal cycle in turn, and examining them to see how confidentiality fits in each for you and your practice. Any ambiguity surrounding confidentiality in the appraisal scheme, and particularly the appraisal interview, will adversely affect the outcomes and therefore the value of the appraisal interview. It is very difficult for people to talk freely and openly if they are unclear as to what will be confidential to the parties concerned and what will be revealed to others. For instance, in an individual interview an appraisee may feel able to share some personal concerns and worries with the appraiser on the assumption that it will be kept confidential between them. If they then discover that all partners and some staff are aware of those private matters, there is little likelihood that they will feel emboldened to seek such support again. A valuable part of the benefit of the protected time of the appraisal interview will thus be lost, let alone any damage done to partner relationships.

The issue of confidentiality will raise its head very early on in any appraisal process, most notably during the following stages.

Before the interview

Part of how you will prepare for appraisal interviews will be collating, scrutinising and screening information gleaned from others. This may be in a formal structure of 360° Appraisal (*see* Step 3) or more informally in discussions with others with whom the appraisee works or liaises.

The question, therefore, at this stage lies in the confidentiality both of the information given to the appraiser, and of the identity of the source. For instance:

- will comments made about the appraisee in this preparatory stage be reported verbatim to the appraisee?

- will the identity of the person(s) making the comment be revealed or anonymised?

You need to think about and plan for the effect on the appraisee of either attributing or anonymising the sources of information.

During the individual or group interview

You need to lay down clear ground rules as to what types of information will remain within the appraisal room, and what will be revealed to others not directly involved in the interview, particularly in relation to any folder being produced for revalidaton.

Appraisal interviews, particularly one-to-one interviews, often facilitate the disclosure of sensitive issues. Understanding that strictly personal issues remain within the interview room needs to be made explicit. Occasionally, however, information given by an appraisee may have significant implications for the practice. Where this occurs, the appraiser must be given the authority by the scheme's rules to act upon such information. For example, if one of your partners informs you that a colleague is abusing drugs or alcohol, or is defrauding the practice, then clearly the confidentiality agreement cannot extend to this type of information. You can deal with this in the rules by giving clear examples of the sort of issues that could override confidentiality constraints. They are likely to be fairly obvious ones.

Similarly, if during the interview it becomes clear that the appraisee is describing actions or omissions which give cause for concern about their fitness to practise, then these too need to be addressed outside the appraisal process. It would be futile to continue with the appraisal interview. In such circumstances the interview needs to be stopped and the matter addressed through the proper channels. This is the same situation as in a managerial hierarchy where the appraisal interview would be stopped if issues of misconduct were revealed. These sorts of situation are less likely to happen in an appraisal interview being carried out by a close colleague and partner, as such concerns are likely to have been brought to light and dealt with in the day-to-day relationships of a practice. If they have not, then some serious thought needs to be given to the way the partnership operates.

Confidentiality and records

Step 9 will give you and your partners the opportunity to decide how to record the appraisal process. Here it is important to refer to the issues of confidentiality that you need to take into account when recording the outcomes of appraisal. For instance, while it is important to record the broad content of an appraisal discussion and to agree it, anxieties about confidentiality will arise if you are seen to be noting every remark. Similarly, it is important that others in your practice can have access to the record of training and development needs that arise in an appraisal, in order to produce an overall training and development plan and thus identify priorities for individuals and the practice overall. The way this part of the form is recorded needs to be sensitive to the need for confidentiality for the individual, and the wider purpose and needs of the practice.

Last, you need to agree as a practice on the security of any appraisal record or records. The following questions can arise:

- where are the records to be kept?

- how many copies of the records will be made?

- how long should the records be retained?

- who can access them?

- if you have a rotating system of one partner leading on appraisal in turn each year, will next year's appraiser have access to this year's record?

- will appraisal records be used as part of the individual's reference should they wish to leave the practice and/or apply for other posts?

Tool 5 is a checklist to help your discussions in this area. You may find it helpful to consolidate your discussion of this tool by putting your answers together in writing to form a clear agreement on confidentiality.

Tool 5 Confidentiality discussion checklist

Preparing for the interview

1 Will we consult others when gathering information about the appraisee?

2 How will this information be revealed to the appraisee – verbatim or will it be 'screened' by the appraiser?

3 Will the people being consulted in this exercise remain anonymous?

4 If so, why?

5 How will anonymity be guaranteed?

6 If the identities of people being consulted are revealed, will they be identified as individuals or as groups of people, e.g. reception staff, nursing team?

7 If the latter, then how will the information gleaned be categorised under each team heading?

During the interview

8 What categories of information will remain confidential to the parties involved in the interview and why?

9 What categories of information will be revealed to others and why?

10 How will we deal with any strictly personal information revealed?

11 How will we deal with information revealed, which has a significant impact on the practice?

Records

12 Who will be responsible for the appraisal record(s)?

13 Where will they be kept?

14 How many copies will be made of the appraisal record?

15 Who will have access to the record?

16 In what circumstances will access be given?

17 How will we deal with breaches of confidentiality?

Step 6 Administering the scheme

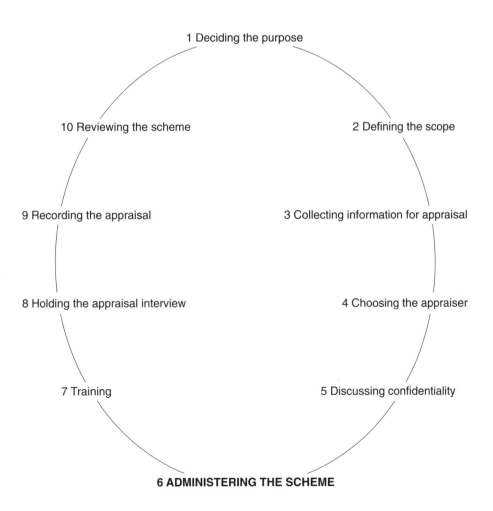

1 Deciding the purpose

10 Reviewing the scheme

2 Defining the scope

9 Recording the appraisal

3 Collecting information for appraisal

8 Holding the appraisal interview

4 Choosing the appraiser

7 Training

5 Discussing confidentiality

6 ADMINISTERING THE SCHEME

Step 6 Administering the scheme

Deciding the content and process of peer appraisal for your practice is the most difficult part of the preparation for appraisal. However, it is also very important to pay attention to the organisational details that underpin successful appraisal. The main questions to be addressed in this respect are:

- where should the appraisal interviews be held?
- how frequently should the interviews occur?
- how long should the interviews take?
- who will organise the structure of the interviews and the overall running of the appraisal process, including producing the documentation?

Where should the appraisal interviews be held?

It is important to make sure that the time given for appraisal is truly protected, free from any interruptions. It is very difficult to concentrate and participate in an appraisal interview if, at the same time, you are worried that you may have to go out on an urgent call. If you opt for group interviews, you will have to consider closing the practice for a half-day, and using locums or a deputising service to

cover. To overcome the expense and disruption of this, some practices have opted for an evening session fuelled by food and refresh-
ment. However, as you will see in Step 8, on handling the actual
appraisal discussion, a balance needs to be kept between being relaxed
and an over-convivial atmosphere which may prevent a full and frank
discussion.

How frequently should appraisals occur?

A clear timetable for the meetings needs to be agreed as well as the
frequency of the appraisal cycle. It needs to be frequent enough to
maintain a dialogue about performance, but not too often to diminish
its importance and make its preparation too much of a chore. It is
important to leave a long enough interval for change to happen as a
result of the previous appraisal, and for development and training
agreed to have demonstrable effect. The most common frequency is
once a year.

How long should the interviews take?

If you have opted for a one-to-one process, then the length of the
interview will be more manageable and predictable than if a number of
partners have to free themselves from other commitments to attend.
The length will also be determined by the design of the appraisal
scheme. There may be significant numbers of areas to be covered, as
you have seen in Step 2 when you decided what to appraise. At least an
hour is realistic. Anything less does not give time in both the individual
and group models for the pleasantries and practicalities to take place
before moving on to the substance of the interview, covering in depth
the agendas of all parties.

Who will organise the process?

The structure of the interview timetable and the overall running of the appraisal process, including producing the documentation, needs care and attention. In most practices, one person probably needs to take overall control of the organisational details − this may be the practice manager. These organisational details will involve:

- timetabling the interviews and ensuring that people are free to attend through hiring locums, rearranging surgeries etc.

- reminding participants of their appointments and ensuring they have the appropriate preparatory paperwork/guidelines etc.

- providing an interview environment conducive to the aims of the scheme

- ensuring that a record of the interview is made soon after the interview and kept according to the agreed rules on confidentiality

- co-ordinating the identification of learning and educational needs with the production and implementation of personal and practice development plans.

Tool 6 is designed to help you and your practice work through the administrative issues, which have to be organised before and after the interview takes place. When you and your practice have answered all these questions, together they could form a short *Note of Guidance* for everyone concerned in the process, so that the administrative process is clear to all and the responsibilities of the administrator are agreed.

Tool 6   Administrative essentials

Before the first interview

- Start and closing date of appraisal process agreed.

- For group interviews, the structure and timing agreed.

- Staff member(s) responsible for the scheme administration, identified and briefed.

- Timetable of interviews agreed and participants informed (and later reminded) of date, time and place.

- Interview preparation forms (*see* Tools 8.1 and 8.2) photocopied and distributed.

- Appraisal record form (*see* Step 9) typed and distributed.

- Action plan forms (*see* Tool 8.6) and PDP forms typed and distributed.

- Confidentiality agreement forms (where used) typed and distributed.

- Room(s) booked and checked.

- Refreshments organised.

- In-house or locum cover organised, surgery times altered and patients informed if necessary.

After the interview

- Reports and action plans collected as agreed.

- Follow up appraisal meeting (if applicable) timetabled.

- Reports and plans sent to relevant people as agreed.

- Development plans collated to inform the practice development plan (*see* Step 9).

- Development plans costed and budgeted.

Step 7 Training for appraisal

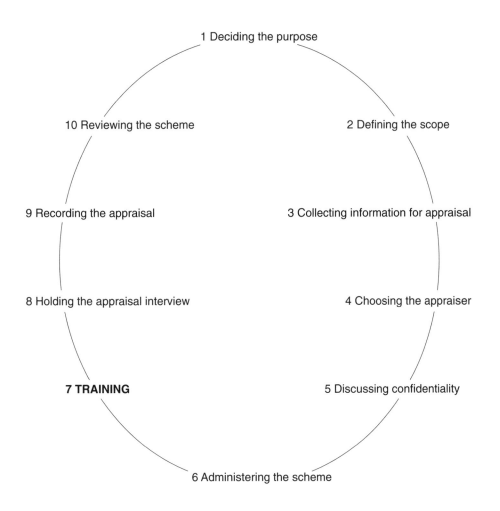

1 Deciding the purpose

10 Reviewing the scheme

2 Defining the scope

9 Recording the appraisal

3 Collecting information for appraisal

8 Holding the appraisal interview

4 Choosing the appraiser

7 TRAINING

5 Discussing confidentiality

6 Administering the scheme

Step 7 Training for appraisal

The whole process of introducing appraisal is of itself a developmental and learning process. Step 8 describes, in detail, the structure of an appraisal interview and the types of issues that can arise. The skills of an appraiser involved in conducting a successful interview are similar to those involved in undertaking a consultation with a patient, though of course it is important to remember the different roles of the appraiser and appraisee and not slip into 'doctor–patient' mode.

This handbook equips general practitioners with the knowledge and insight needed to introduce and implement peer appraisal. Clearly, working through this handbook is in itself a good learning process and enhances awareness of gaps in knowledge and skills. Some may feel as a result that they require no further training. However for others, this section, Step 7, seeks to highlight specific training needs for those with little or no experience in some of the key areas, or those seeking greater confidence, through training, to undertake an appraisal interview.

Approaching an appraisal interview with confidence and handling it successfully involves a combination of knowledge, insight and skill. Knowledge and insight comes from an understanding of appraisal and the aims and details of your practice's scheme.

Reading about a subject, however, may not equip you on its own with the skills to undertake a peer appraisal interview, particularly one where difficult issues have to be tackled. You must decide what further training, if any, you need to enable you to undertake this sensitive and sophisticated meeting between two peers. Box 7 outlines the skills involved in undertaking a successful appraisal interview. By reading this chapter and then using the proforma set out in Tool 7, you will be able to assess whether or not you are equipped to handle this successfully and whether you would benefit from training. You and your practice can then discuss the most appropriate way of meeting these training needs.

Tool 7   Identifying appraisal skills

Skill needed	Already present	Training needed	Likely source
Establishing a good rapport	☐	☐	....
Raising sensitive issues	☐	☐	....
Assertiveness	☐	☐	....
Confidence	☐	☐	....
Facilitation	☐	☐	....
Constructive feedback	☐	☐	....
Empathy	☐	☐	....
Questioning	☐	☐	....

Box 7   The key skills involved in appraisal interviews

For both parties

- Establishing rapport and a relaxed atmosphere.

- Tackling difficult and/or sensitive issues. The aim here is to raise an issue in such a way that it can be discussed calmly and maturely without defensiveness or aggression being invoked. The aim is to get a constructive outcome, where the problem can be tackled and moved forward, with all parties maintaining respect for each other and feeling that things have progressed.

- Being assertive and not aggressive.

- Retaining independence and not being pressurised into unrealistic commitments, for example expending practice resources (particularly time) or agreements to change behaviour which are not possible.

For the appraiser

- Facilitating self-appraisal through skilful questions and reflection, enabling the appraisee to identify accurately their own strengths and weaknesses, training and development needs and areas which they need to change and the strategies involved in doing this.

- Giving constructive feedback on the appraisee's performance and contribution to the partnership and the wider primary healthcare team. Step 8 gives further details in this area.

- Helping your colleagues to express their concerns, hopes and fears about anything that concerns, directly or indirectly, their work and the practice.

When you have identified any skills or experience in which you feel you would benefit from tutoring or training, then finding the right tutor and/or course is crucial. A GP Tutor or someone already trained may be right for you. However, if you opt for a course always scrutinise a course programme to ensure that it fits your needs. A course where numbers are restricted implies that tutoring is on an individual or small group basis – the best environment for learning appraisal skills. Also, courses which are geared to practising appraisal interviewing techniques using role plays, case studies and video playback, indicate that the training is focused on the skills required to undertake an appraisal interview. *See* p. 121 for some suggestions as to ways of going about finding an appropriate way forward.

However, do not feel restricted to a traditional appraisal course. Depending on the training needs you have identified from Tool 7, an assertiveness course or a course on giving effective feedback may well be appropriate to your needs as an addition to the appraisal course, or as an alternative to it. Constructive feedback is such a crucially important topic that we discuss it now in some detail.

Constructive feedback

Whichever type of appraisal – one-to-one or group – the ability to give constructive feedback is a key skill that needs to be both identified and acquired if it is missing. It will often be the determining factor in the success or otherwise of the appraisal interview and the reputation of the scheme. Much depends on it, as the potential for damage, both to individuals and the integrity of the scheme, is significant.

In addition to the appraisal setting, feedback occurs in many areas of our lives – in everyday communications with people reacting to what we have said or done, on training courses and from ourselves reflecting on how we feel about the things we do. Feedback from others in our professional lives is essential for anybody who wishes to develop and grow. It gives us the opportunity to change the way we do things and the more confident among us actively seek it. Equally, such people provide comments in a way which enhances performance and relationships.

What is constructive feedback?

John Thatcher in an article in *Training and Development (UK)* has defined constructive feedback as:

> 'information about performance or behaviour that leads to an action to affirm or develop that performance or behaviour.'

This definition assumes that feedback is constructive and is about building on what is positive and planning further development.

Constructive feedback is the process whereby a link is established between what a person does and says and understanding the impact these have on others. In terms of appraisal, it is probably the most important skill you can develop.

Constructive feedback is the characteristic which differentiates between:

- managers who motivate and help their colleagues, and those who struggle in their people-management role

- coaches and advisers who make a real difference in the performance and behaviours of others, and those who just skim the surface

- mentors who release potential, and those who stifle it

- people who make effective team members, and those who hinder team performance

- people who gain real commitment from others to a personal plan for development, and those who elicit merely lip service to change.

The difference between *constructive* feedback and *destructive* criticism

Feedback can be either positive – reinforcing a person's strengths and behaviours – or negative – an attempt to influence a person's weaknesses. Both types of feedback, to be effective, must be constructive. However, in an appraisal interview it is all too easy to gloss over the strengths, to take them for granted, and focus on the weaknesses in such a way that the feedback is unbalanced and becomes destructive. It is important, therefore, to start with positive statements and then move on to the problems, where possible letting the appraisee speak first. In that way constructive feedback can be ensured and negative feedback is cushioned.

Constructive feedback is facilitated by having agreed standards within which behaviour or performance can be discussed with a plan for development. The appraiser therefore needs to consider the following.

- Analyse the problem, disentangling feelings and impressions from facts and objective evidence; this will lead to identifying what needs changing. Ensure you have examples to support your statements.

- Decide on your outcome – what you want to achieve from the discussion – and construct a strategy which will help you to achieve it. However, never forget the option of not raising the issue at all. Occasionally, when preparing to give constructive feedback, it becomes clear that giving the feedback (no matter how constructively) will adversely affect the relationship. This may lead you to conclude that any gains are outweighed by damage to the relationship.

- Think through and anticipate some strategies that can be offered to the appraisee to develop. This ensures that the tone of the discussion is positive and about the future, rather than unpicking the past with no plan for development. This is one of the reasons why identifying the categories of subjects, which will form the content of a peer appraisal interview, is so important, as is having some form of explicit standards. This provides the context within which constructive discussions can take place.

Destructive criticism often occurs when a constructive and professional context, as described above, is missing and takes the form of generalised, subjective comments focusing on personal characteristics and perceived negative attitudes. For example, telling someone that they have a very obstructive attitude towards others can only elicit anger or hurt in the recipient. It will not only fail to gain any change in the person but will damage the relationship between the appraiser and appraisee.

Your tone of voice and body language are crucial in this exercise and must not be under estimated. Positive, well thought through words can be undermined and corrupted by the wrong tone of voice and body language. It is interesting to note that words account for 7% of a message, how the words are spoken (tone of voice, emphasis and pace) account for 38% and body language 55%.

Box 8 gives some examples of opening statements in dealing with problems, each showing a destructive and a constructive approach.

Box 8 Examples of destructive and constructive approaches

1 The problem
The appraisee regularly turns up late for partnership meetings and leaves early pleading another, more important, commitment. The meetings are arranged one month in advance.

Destructive approach:
'I want to discuss your time keeping for the partnership meetings. You're always late. It's very frustrating for the rest of us and we are getting quite fed up with your tardiness and leaving early. Don't you think the meetings are important?'

Constructive approach:
'I would like to talk about how you see the partnership meetings. You have always been very positive about the importance of communication and meetings, but you have difficulty in getting to the partnership ones. Because this seemed odd I have noted what has happened to all of us as far as attendance at meetings is concerned. You may be surprised to know that over the last year you have arrived, on average, 20 minutes late at the start of 10 of the 12 meetings and have left, on average, half an hour before the end in nine of the meetings. This, as you can see from this record, is not true of other partners. I am sure this will concern you as much as it concerns me. Perhaps we could talk the reasons through.'

2 The problem
The practice operates a personal list system. The appraisee is reluctant to use the practice nurses and continues to do her own cervical smears. She also insists on seeing her own diabetic patients whilst the rest of the partners refer them to the nurse run, but doctor supported, diabetic clinic.

Destructive approach:
'We need to talk about a problem we've discussed before – the nurses are very hurt that you don't trust them enough to do the cervical smears or to see your diabetic patients. It's a waste of resources and it is undermining the nurse team. We have to do something about it.'

Constructive approach:
'I'd like to revisit an aspect of practice work, which we have discussed before. It's the relationship between us, the partners, and the nursing team, and the best way we, as a practice, can offer care to our patients, particularly those needing cervical smears and our diabetics. Can we discuss the extra benefits you feel your patients receive from seeing you rather than the nurses?'

3   The problem
The appraisee is regularly rude to staff and despite the practice manager talking to him about this (and the appraiser too has had a word), nothing has changed.

Destructive approach:
'I have to talk to you about the way you treat the staff. I have talked to you about this, the practice manager has talked to you about this and you continue to shout at the receptionists. What is wrong? You do realise we'll end up in an Employment Tribunal if this continues, don't you?'

Constructive approach:
'I would like to discuss our roles as employers of the staff and ways in which we can improve. I know we have discussed this before, and in particular we have talked about your style. The reason I am raising it again is because how we manage the staff has a significant impact on the practice and has legal implications. What are your thoughts?'

Box 9 gives some tips that summarise approaches to constructive feedback.

Box 9   Tips on giving constructive feedback

1   It should be balanced, paying as much, if not more, attention to the appraisee's strengths (with specific examples) as to the appraisee's weaknesses.

2   Analyse any problems you wish to raise, identifying desired outcomes and developing strategies to achieve these.

3   Be objective and stick to facts, with examples, discussing the issue using neutral, non-judgemental language.

4   It should be specific – never make negative generalisations about a person's behaviour or character.

5   It should be realistic. There is little point in addressing personality traits, which cannot be changed; stick to behaviours, which can be modified.

6   It should be consultative where both parties are engaged in discussing the feedback, jointly working through ideas and solutions.

Step 8 Holding the appraisal interview

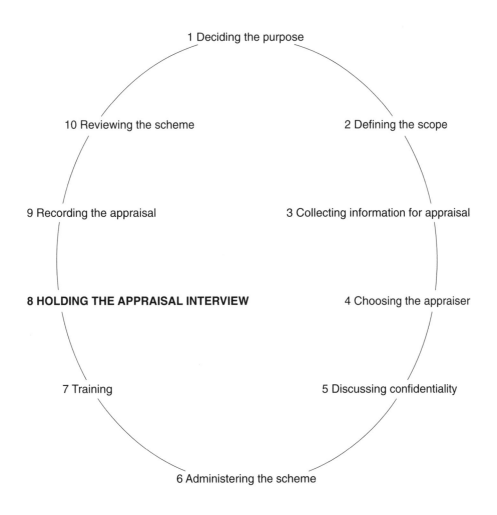

1 Deciding the purpose

10 Reviewing the scheme

2 Defining the scope

9 Recording the appraisal

3 Collecting information for appraisal

8 HOLDING THE APPRAISAL INTERVIEW

4 Choosing the appraiser

7 Training

5 Discussing confidentiality

6 Administering the scheme

Step 8　Holding the appraisal interview

The interview is the heart of the appraisal process. Thorough preparation, working through the steps in this handbook, will help to ensure the process runs smoothly and effectively. The work that you have done so far, both individually and as a practice, will go a long way to ensuring it is a beneficial and supportive process. The next step is to consider how to prepare for and conduct the interview.

Box 10 sets out diagrammatically the processes that are described here.

Box 10　The process of the interview

Action	Tool
Prepare	3.6, 3.7 and 8.2
Open and agree the ground rules	8.3
Agree the agenda	8.4
Raise the issues	8.5
Agree the action	8.6

The appraisee

Preparation

As the appraisee, you will prepare in a similar way for an individual or a group interview. You will certainly gain more from the appraisal process if you have spent some time on self-appraisal and in gathering evidence by some of the methods described in Step 3. In peer appraisal, the appraisee is an equal partner in the appraisal process and thus should see the appraisal interview as an opportunity for self-reflection and analysis. It is vital for a peer appraisal scheme to be viewed as a dynamic process between different key players in the practice, and not something that is 'done to' an appraisee. This cannot happen without a commitment to spending time preparing for the interview.

When you are preparing for appraisal in your practice you need to agree with all concerned on the use of a pre-appraisal form which will allow the appraisee to reflect constructively and appropriately on each of the areas under discussion. Tool 8.1 is an example of a pre-appraisal form which builds on the information you collected in Tools 2.1, 2.2 and 3.10. It may need to be amended to reflect the particular emphasis your practice wishes to place on one competence or area of practice. This is a preparatory document to give confidence in approaching the interview. It can help to organise the information brought to the interview and the evidence being presented, as well as serve as an aide-mémoire during the interview.

Tool 8.1   Sample pre-appraisal form for the appraisee

Name .... Date of interview .... Period covered by the appraisal ....

This form is for you to make notes in preparation for your appraisal meeting. Bearing in mind the areas agreed on in Step 2, draw on any information you may have collected in Step 3. The main areas you listed in Tools 2.2 and 3.9 will be the headings on Part 1 of the form. The information on this form is for you alone and will only be shared with others if you wish to do so.

Part 1

Key areas	What strengths do you demonstrate in this area? With examples and evidence from the past year	What aspects of this area of work have you done less effectively and why? With examples and evidence from the past year	What are your development/training needs in this area?
Good clinical care			
Maintaining good practice			
Good relationships with patients			
Working with colleagues			

Teaching

Research

Personal health

Part 2

What objectives will you set yourself for the next 12 months?

What support will you need from the practice and from individuals to achieve this?

The appraiser

One-to-one interviews

Preparation

The appraiser should use a pre-appraisal proforma similar to that used by the appraisee (Tool 8.1). A sample is given as Tool 8.2.

It is essential in any appraisal interview that the appraisee has confidence in the skill and integrity of the appraiser. This is even more important for peer appraisal, particularly concerning any problematic issues which the appraiser wishes to address. Ensuring that such sensitive issues are handled constructively and assertively requires thorough preparation.

The appraiser should gather evidence on the appraisee's performance using some of the tools described in Step 3. It is important that appraisal interviews are not dependent on evidence collected in the two weeks before the due date, but be based on a data collection process that continues all the year. Otherwise the interview will tend to focus on only the most recent events. The better the preparation the more likely that sensitive and problematic areas will be addressed constructively and assertively.

Tool 8.2 Sample pre-appraisal form for the appraiser(s)

Name of appraisee .... Name of appraiser(s) ....
Date of interview .... Period covered by the appraisal ....

Bearing in mind the areas agreed in Step 2, use whatever information you have collected in Step 3 to complete this tool prior to the appraisal meeting.

Part 1

Key areas	What strengths does the appraisee demonstrate in this area? With examples and evidence from the past year	What aspects of this area of work has the appraisee done less effectively and why? With examples and evidence from the past year	What are the appraisee's development/training needs in this area?
Good clinical care			
Maintaining good practice			
Good relationships with patients			
Working with colleagues			

Teaching

Research

Personal health

Part 2

What objectives might you set for the appraisee for the next 12 months?

What support will the appraisee need from the practice and from individuals to achieve this?

Opening the interview

Your first aim as an appraiser is to relax the appraisee, as he/she must be able to make full use of this opportunity to reflect objectively on successes and failures. Your competence as an appraiser and as a willing mentor is crucial to this process. Establishing rapport and allowing the appraisee to both reflect on the past year and express their hopes and plans for the future are fundamental to the interview's success. It is sometimes the most difficult part of the process, and it is worth thinking about carefully in advance. Tool 8.3 gives some suggestions for opening gambits.

Tool 8.3 Ideas for opening appraisal interviews

Purpose of the interview:
'This is our opportunity to take some protected time out to discuss your work in the practice, the practice itself and to look at your personal development needs over the next year. I see myself as a willing mentor. After all, this is your interview, not mine, and my role is to facilitate your analysis of the past year and give balanced constructive feedback.'

Agreeing the agenda:
'This is time I very much value, the opportunity to reflect on what has happened over the last year. We will of course be following the topics on the appraisal form. We may both have some additional areas to discuss – do you have any you want to add now? Here are mine.'

Recognising past difficulties:
'I am so glad we have got this opportunity to sit down in peace and discuss the very traumatic/difficult time we have had recently in the practice. More importantly, I see this as a way of putting recent events into perspective. So many other good things have happened over the last year and perhaps we could start by examining those before we move on to the more problematic issues. What do you think?'

A new partner/assistant:
'You will have received the guidance notes on our peer appraisal scheme and we have talked about it recently. Before we start on the interview proper, what are your views on the scheme itself and what would you like to gain from this meeting?'

A partner who is leaving/retiring soon:
'I know you are leaving the practice soon and therefore perhaps the discussions about your future and your personal development plan may be redundant. I do think, however, that meeting like this will be very beneficial, especially for the practice and me! I think it's a great opportunity to get a perspective, from someone with your experience, of the strengths and weaknesses of the practice as a whole. Also, it would be very useful to get your initial thoughts on recruiting for your replacement and any internal structural changes you think we should make at this time.'

Individuals are far more committed to a line of action if they themselves have suggested it. Therefore, it is desirable for the appraisee to appraise him/herself and to suggest ways of improving or building on current strengths and interests. The interview, therefore, should not be focused on you as the appraiser telling, but rather you should concentrate on encouraging the appraisee to assess his/her own strengths and weaknesses, and to come up with ideas on improving performance and identifying development needs.

Conducting the interview

The shape of the interview may depend on the issues to be discussed, but you might like to agree a common framework to ensure a consistent and fair approach between different colleagues. Tool 8.4 is a form that can be used by the appraiser(s) to set the agenda for the interview.

The main principles of good appraising mirror those of patient-centred consulting. These would include:

- beginning each new section with an open question

- asking for clarification and examples as necessary

- being aware of verbal and non-verbal cues, particularly words suggesting anxiety or stress, or where non-verbal signals seem to contradict the verbal message

- encouraging evidence wherever possible to illustrate and back up opinions

- summarising your interpretations back to the appraisee to make sure that you have been accurate in what you have heard

- using the rules of 'good feedback' as set out in Step 7.

It is, however, very important to remember that this is not a patient consultation, and both the appraiser and the appraisee must not drop into the doctor–patient role, otherwise the whole benefit of peer appraisal is lost. It can become a teaching or counselling session, not getting to grips with the difficult areas of concern to one or both.

It is also important to be prepared to address difficult and sensitive areas, and Tool 8.5 is an exercise that will enable you to plan the opening gambits for approaching tricky issues. It also gives some practice in responding to difficult appraisee openings!

Tool 8.4   Sample appraisal interview agenda

CONFIDENTIAL

Name ....
Date of qualification ....
Period covered by the interview ....
Date of interview ....
Appraisers' names and titles ....
....

1   Effective areas of work during the year?

2   Less effective areas of work?

3   Developmental needs to be discussed?

4   Possible targets for the next year?

5   Means of reviewing the targets?

6   Objectives for the next 12 months?

7   Support needed from the practice and from individuals?

Tool 8.5   Raising sensitive issues

What opening questions would you use to raise the following issues with the appraisee?

1   The reasons behind a pattern of mistakes or oversights which have occurred recently.

2   The failure of the appraisee to adhere to partnership decisions.

3   The appraisee is extremely sympathetic to staff and his/her 'open door' policy to employees is now undermining the practice manager's position.

4   The failure of the appraisee to use his computer consistently for data entry, thus corrupting the practice's audit programme.

5   The appraisee's view of the support you and your other partners offer him/her.

6   The appraisee's perceptions of his/her own weaknesses.

How would you respond to the following statements made by an appraisee?

7   'Well, actually, I don't believe in this type of appraisal anyway.'

8   'Totally confidentially, absolutely between you and me, I want to alert you to ...'

9   'Well, actually, I don't find you very supportive. You and the other partners rarely agree with any of my suggestions.'

10   'I really enjoy working here but I am having problems with the practice nurses who think too much of themselves and don't seem to have any respect for us doctors.'

Closing the interview

It is important at the end of the interview to agree targets and objectives with timescales and follow-up dates. Whilst discussing the appraisee's training and development needs and how these will be fed into his/her personal development plan, ensure that you are not committing the practice to an educational expense (either in terms of money or time out of the practice) which cannot be afforded.

The planned time schedule of the interview should be adhered to as closely as possible, though not slavishly. Sometimes crucial and occasionally emotional areas can be touched on, and they need space and time to resolve. This may be by extending the interview to explore them in more depth, or by ensuring they are acknowledged and that other sources of help are suggested and agreed.

Having said that, both the appraiser and appraisee should make sure they are aware of the passage of time, although the onus is probably more on the appraiser to structure the interviews according to the agreed timescale. It is important, however, that significant issues are not ignored because of the pressure of time.

The concluding few minutes of the interview should be spent summarising the findings in all areas of the agenda and making sure the appraiser and appraisee's interpretation are the same, or if they are not, record only this as the case. Additionally, the main outcomes must be agreed in line with the sample action plan set out as Tool 8.6.

It will need to be made clear to the appraisee in this individual interview that any identified personal development needs may not be a priority in terms of practice development, and no promises or commitments should be entered into. When all appraisals are completed the overall training needs against the practice development plan will need to be discussed as a group, to decide on the priorities that the practice feels able to support.

Tool 8.6 Appraisal action plan

Name ....

Date of appraisal interview ....

1 The following objectives and targets have been agreed for the following year:

    ....
    ....
    ....

2 To achieve them the appraisee needs to:

    ....
    ....
    ....

3 The other partner(s)/practice team etc. [identify who] needs to:

    ....
    ....

4 The following training, educational, development and/or experience needs have been identified:

    ....
    ....

5 Our next meeting, if applicable, to discuss and/or review this action plan will take place on ....

This Action Plan is a 'live' document and will be kept and should be referred to by the appraisee throughout the year.

Group interviews

If the partnership has opted for a group-based interview process, the first key decision to be made is whether one doctor, the lead appraiser, can organise the whole system, run the meetings, record the outcomes and appraise. Some people may feel confident in doing this. Alternatively, the doctors may decide that there should be an external facilitator. *See* p. 125 for some suggestions on filling this role – the important thing is that the person should be skilled and experienced in facilitation. Sometimes, the practice manager is able to fill this role providing they have the necessary training and experience.

Preparation

This stage differs from that for individual interviews. Running a group process requires different but complementary skills. In particular, the timing needs to be planned in detail beforehand and made explicit to all participants.

In group peer appraisal meetings, feedback is gathered more widely. Staff and nursing feedback can be elicited and collated in an anonymous way by the practice. Again, the practice manager could do this if there is an appropriate relationship of trust and maturity between practice manager and the rest of the practice, and if he/she is prepared to take on this sensitive task. Tools 3.6 and 3.7 in Step 3 may help in this.

Additionally, the partners themselves have an important role to play in providing feedback to each other – one of the strengths (and threats) of peer appraisal. It is useful for the doctors not only to complete their own feedback from Tool 8.2 but also to make brief feedback notes about each of their colleagues using copies of Tool 3.6, the team feedback questionnaire.

Running the group interview process

Opening the meeting

The successful outcome of a peer appraisal group meeting is highly dependent on how well the meeting is run. It is the role of the group facilitator (or lead general practitioner appraiser if that is the same person) to set the 'scene' and lay down the ground rules for the conduct of the meeting. These would include:

- sticking to the agreed timetable – plan to give a doctor at least half an hour, preferably an hour

- observing confidentiality concerning any issues raised in the meeting (except in the unlikely event of serious health issues or dangerous practice being unexpectedly raised)

- allowing colleagues time to speak without interruption

- observing the rules of giving feedback, especially in terms of constructive criticism aimed at behaviours that are amenable to change.

Conducting the meeting

A formal structure to the meeting is important, especially in the first few cycles of peer appraisal group sessions. It may well be that in large practices, if this method of appraisal is used, several meetings will be needed, or several sub-groups of partners agreed.

The lead appraiser/facilitator needs to ask each doctor in turn to present the main points from their self-appraisal (Tool 8.1), which should be backed up with some evidence using a selection of the tools and methods described in Step 3. The rest of the group can then add their comments, tailored to address the specific areas of strengths and concerns raised by the doctor being appraised, to define the key issues to be addressed. You can then start the group discussion.

When the appraisee's allotted time (say, 30 minutes per individual) is drawing to a close the lead appraiser/facilitator should summarise the key points that have been raised, and check these with the appraisee. The group then should agree the action points which will go into the individual development plan, and list the priorities for the practice development plan.

This cycle should be repeated for all the doctors. If there is no facilitator, another doctor must take on this role whilst the lead appraiser is being appraised.

Closing the meeting

The meeting should not be allowed to run over the allocated time. Once the cycle has been completed for all doctors, the main action points for the personal and practice development plans are reiterated and the meeting brought to a close. Each doctor is responsible for completing his or her own action plans and providing a copy for the lead appraiser. Further details on translating the outcomes of appraisal into a personal development plan are given in Step 9.

Step 9 Recording the appraisal

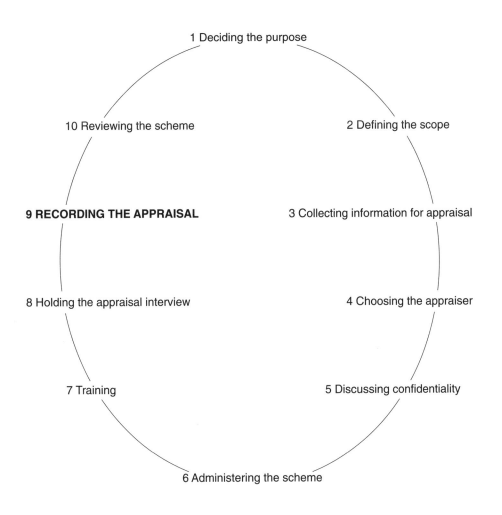

1 Deciding the purpose

10 Reviewing the scheme

2 Defining the scope

9 RECORDING THE APPRAISAL

3 Collecting information for appraisal

8 Holding the appraisal interview

4 Choosing the appraiser

7 Training

5 Discussing confidentiality

6 Administering the scheme

Step 9   Recording the appraisal

For most interviews a record needs to be kept, under each category, of the main points raised with any agreements and future plans agreed. However, it makes little sense, and indeed can impede the flow and value of any appraisal interview, if a record is made of every remark and discussion in the interview itself.

Many appraisal schemes will have, as one of its purposes, the identification of the doctor's learning and educational needs. In order for this information to be transferred to the doctor's and the practice's development plans, these development needs have to be shared with others.

This is not an issue for group interviews when part of the group process requires agreement on key outcomes for each doctor. These become the basis of each individual's development plan, which is understood and approved by all the practice doctors. Appraisal systems based on individual interviews may need to have a group meeting when the suggested outcomes and training plans of individual doctors are discussed and agreed by the group.

Personal development plans

Identifying the professional development needs of people is a fundamental aim of most appraisal schemes. As we stated in the beginning, the government, the public and the medical profession itself now clearly recognise the need for ongoing professional education and performance review that is explicit and externally monitored. The importance of training and development has shifted from the didactic to the facilitative, with doctors now being asked to be much more active in identifying their own learning needs and planning their own training and professional development. Personal and practice development plans will be required for all doctors as part of the external appraisal and revalidation process. Peer appraisal carried out using individual and group interviews can lead on to the development of personal and practice plans. The tools and methods in Step 3, particularly Tool 3.10, can all be used to identify educational needs. The appraisal interview is a useful forum for discussing and refining these needs and agreeing strategies to meet them. This is the basic process whereby education and development plans are written.

There are a variety of guidelines available on how each doctor should set about writing his/her own personal development plan (*see* p. 122). The main elements of all plans are the identification of needs, the actions needed to meet them (which will have been done in the appraisal process) and the setting of a specific time framework. Tool 9 is the framework for a personal development plan based on the work you have already undertaken. Use Tools 3.10, 8.1 and 8.6 to help in this task.

Tool 9 A personal development plan

Doctor .... Date ....

Key areas	Educational needs	How identified	Means of addressing needs	Outcomes/evidence	Timescale
1 Good clinical care					
2 Maintaining good practice					
3 Good relationships with patients					
4 Working with colleagues					
5 Teaching					
6 Research					
7 Personal health					

The production of personal development plans owned by the individual and shared with the group is a rewarding process. Developing an organisational culture, which values personal development, brings benefit to everyone and this process can readily be extended to all core members of the primary care team. Receptionist and nursing staff can use most of the processes of peer appraisal described in this book. Setting up a robust peer appraisal system for doctors prepares the ground for the extension of this to the whole team, and the production of a practice development plan truly owned by all the team members.

Step 10 Reviewing the scheme

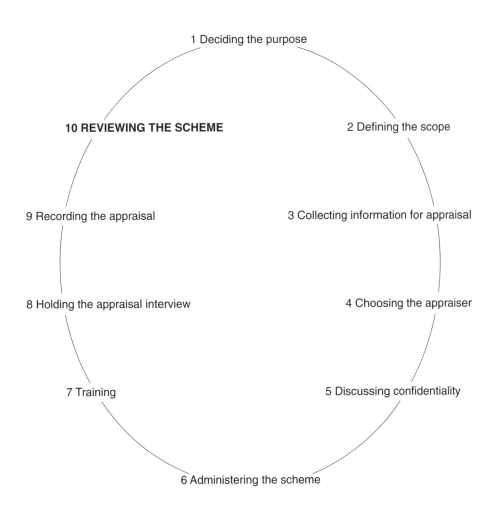

1 Deciding the purpose

10 REVIEWING THE SCHEME

2 Defining the scope

9 Recording the appraisal

3 Collecting information for appraisal

8 Holding the appraisal interview

4 Choosing the appraiser

7 Training

5 Discussing confidentiality

6 Administering the scheme

Step 10 Reviewing the scheme

When a scheme has been firmly established, it should be reviewed about every three years. However, when a scheme is first introduced closer monitoring should take place. Large organisations involving large numbers of people can afford the luxury of a pilot scheme. Practices, and particularly with the numbers involved in peer appraisal, are simply not big enough to pilot a scheme before 'going live'. It is important, therefore, to take stock fairly soon after the scheme's introduction, once the last of the peer appraisal interviews has taken place. The longer-term review of a new scheme should occur at about 18 months after its introduction. Tool 10.1 is a checklist for the short-term review, which should be conducted with all the partners soon after the interviews have been completed. Tool 10.2 is the checklist for the longer-term evaluation, and should be conducted about 18 months after the scheme's introduction.

All participants should be involved in both the short- and long-term evaluations and the results of these questionnaires listed in Tools 10.1 and 10.2 should form the basis of discussions and modifications to the scheme, if appropriate.

Tool 10.1   The short-term review by participants: to be completed after the first round of appraisal interviews/meetings has taken place

Before the interview
Briefing/training received:
1   Was it understandable?
2   Was it pitched at the right level?
3   Did it cover the appropriate areas?
4   Were the methods used and time allowed appropriate?
5   Did it help you understand the scheme?
6   Did it prepare you adequately for the interview?

Collecting information:
7   How much time did you spend collecting information prior to the interview?
8   How useful was this information to the appraisal interview?
9   Did you encounter any problems in this information-gathering exercise?

Completing the preparation form (if applicable):
10   Was it understandable?
11   Did it cover the appropriate areas?
12   How much time did you spend on completing it?
13   How helpful was it to the interview?
14   How did you use the preparation form?

The interview
15   Was the interview delayed at all – if so, by how long?
16   How long did the interview last?
17   How useful was it in achieving [insert main purpose of scheme]?
18   How useful was it as an opportunity to exchange views?
19   Has there been any change in the relationship between you and [insert name of colleague/s involved in the interview]?
20   What knowledge and insight did you gain as a result of the appraisal process?

After the interview
21   Describe your feelings after the interview.
22   How long after the interview did you complete/have sight of (as applicable) the appraisal record?

Tool 10.2   The longer-term review

Longer-term review by participants

1   What training and development has resulted from your appraisal interview?

2   How satisfied are you with your personal development plan?

3   Has the appraisal interview been followed up with meetings to discuss the action plan/personal development plan etc.?

4   Overall, how satisfied are you with the scheme and what suggestions do you have to improve it?

Appendix

Additional sources and tools for collecting evidence for appraisal

Self-administered tests

Multiple choice questions

There is good evidence that we do not accurately identify gaps in our knowledge. A recent study showed that doctors' own assessment of their strengths and weaknesses did not correlate closely with objective testing. MCQs are reckoned to be the most objective way of checking clinical knowledge at a theoretical level. They are less good at testing specific skills, decision making and attitudes

Test scores of MCQs can be compared and shared with colleagues, thus defining areas where a practice-based educational initiative would be useful and appropriate. The RCGP publishes MCQ tests in 14 key subject areas (*see* p. 124).

Confidence rating scales

These are much more subjective and may not accurately reflect the doctor's true knowledge base. However, they may be helpful in identifying specific areas of weakness, as perceived by the appraisee, and comparing these with feedback from team colleagues who may differ in their assessment.

There are a range of scales available, most of which have been developed to help plan an individualised training programme for general practice registrars. A good example is the Northumbria Vocational Training Scheme Rating Scale (*see* p. 124).

Clinical audit

Many areas of clinical activity can be evaluated using audit skills and drawing on the increasingly widely available evidence-based guidelines for a range of conditions. If one doctor is individually responsible for a specific clinical area such as ante-natal care or diabetes, part of his or her appraisal might include completing the audit cycle relating to an aspect of patient care in these areas.

In a group practice without personal lists audit may more accurately reflect practice performance than individual effort. However, if you are in a practice where the doctors use the computer for data entry in the consultation, it may be possible to compare the clinical recording of different doctors for specific conditions. It may be a particularly important tool in single-handed practice. Here it can be used to demonstrate high-quality care in a range of clinical conditions such as asthma, diabetes and ischaemic heart disease, where regional or national guidelines are in place.

The basic process of audit is reproduced opposite, using ischaemic heart disease as the exemplar.

Example of an audit cycle

1   How many of my patients with known ischaemic heart disease are taking aspirin?
     Action – do computer search.
2   How many should be?
     Action – look at local guidelines, contraindications and so on.
3   Intervention if necessary.
     Action – increase use of aspirin by writing to or reviewing all patients not taking aspirin who should be; improve recording in the notes.
4   Repeat Stage 1 to see if any improvement has been achieved.

Audit can also be used to review non-clinical aspects of practice activity such as availability of appointments, telephone access, doctor's time-keeping, missing records etc. These may provide useful objective evidence for discussion at the appraisal meeting.

Clinical activity

Other aspects of clinical activity can also be reasonably easily re-viewed as a prelude to the peer appraisal meeting, especially if the appraisee identifies a specific need in a particular area. Two examples are given below.

Referrals

Referral rates are known to vary considerably both within and between practices. You can obtain computerised data on referrals from hospitals and discuss the reasons for variations. These may be supplemented by review of a range of 'real' or specimen cases. Significant variations from the practice 'mean' need to be explained and educational needs defined, which may also be brought to the appraisal meeting.

Prescribing

Most health authorities have certain prescribing guidelines, which 'benchmark' good prescribing practice. These provide a good starting point for discussing variations in prescribing rates within a partnership. Again, if you identify big deviations from the mean you will need to address them. PACT data can be useful especially for drugs prescribed acutely such as antibiotics. In some areas practices have shared data such as on a PCG-wide basis. As you will discover, important educational needs can emerge from this process.

Case analysis

This is a process widely used in registrar teaching. It provides a forum for exploring a range of issues which may arise in a consultation, including:

- defining the problems presented in the consultation

- discussing management and any alternative strategies

- exploring the doctor's feelings about the consultation.

Case analysis can be a very powerful tool for exploring both clinical diagnosis and management issues and non-clinical issues such as management of time, recognition of stress in one's self, plus the appropriate use of primary care team colleagues. A seemingly simple case picked randomly from a surgery can provide a rich source of information for debate, as can complex patients selected by the doctor for discussion. Given the length of time available for the appraisal interview, ideally case analysis should take place between appraisal meetings, and the outcomes and educational needs brought to the appraisal meeting for discussion.

Further information and suggested reading

Formal public documents

Department of Health

- *Clinical Governance: Quality in the new NHS* (1998)
- *A First Class Service: Quality in the new NHS* (1998)
- *Supporting Doctors, Protecting Patients* (1999)
- *An Organisation with Memory* (2000)
- *The NHS Plan* (England) (2000)
- *Confidence in the Future for Patients* (2000)

These and other Department of Health publications are available free on request from the relevant Government Office.

Department of Health for England
Richmond House
79 Whitehall
London SW1A 2NL
Tel: 0207 210 3000
www.doh.gov.uk

Scottish Executive
St Andrew's House
Edinburgh EH1 3DG
Tel: 0131 556 8400
Fax: 0131 244 8240

email: ceu@scotland.gov.uk
www.scotland.gov.uk

The National Assembly for Wales
Cardiff Bay
Cardiff CF99 1NA
Tel: 029 2082 5111

email: assembly.info@wales.gsi.gov.uk

Northern Ireland Assembly
Castle Building
Stormont
Belfast BS4

email: info.office@niassembly.gov.uk
www.ni-assembly.gov.uk

Royal College of General Practitioners

- *Good Medical Practice for General Practitioners* (2000)

RCGP Publications Department
14 Princes Gate
London SW7 1PM
Tel: 0207 581 3232

or on their website: www.rcgp.org.uk

General Medical Council

- *Good Medical Practice* (1998)
- *Revalidating Doctors: Ensuring standards, securing the future* (1999)

External Relations Office
General Medical Council
178 Great Portland Street
London W1N 6JE
Tel: 0207 915 3507
Fax: 0207 915 3685

or via the website: www.gmc-uk.org

Books, reports and articles

On appraisal

- Haman H and Irvine S (2001) *Good People, Good Practice: A practical guide to managing personnel in the new primary care organisations.* Radcliffe Medical Press, Oxford.

- BAMM (1999) *Appraisal in Action: Appraisal for hospital doctors.* British Association of Medical Managers, Stockport.

- SCOPME (1996) *Appraising Doctors and Dentists in Training.* Standing Committee on Post Graduate Medical and Dental Education, London.

- Edis M (1995) *Performance Management and Appraisal in Health Services.* Kogan Page, London.

- Thatcher J (1994) Motivating people via feedback. *Training and Development (UK).* **12**(7): 8–10, 12.

- Mehrabian A and Ferris I (1967) Inference of attitudes from non-verbal communication in two channels. *Journal of Counselling Psychology.* **31**: 248–52.

- Jelley D and van Zwanenberg T (2000) Peer appraisal in general practice: a descriptive study in the Northern Deanery. *Education for General Practice.* **11**: 281–7.

On continuing professional development and development plans

- Wakley G, Chambers R and Field S (2000) *Continuing Professional Development in Primary Care: Making it happen.* Radcliffe Medical Press, Oxford.

- Rughani A (2000) *The GP's Guide to Personal Development Plans.* Radcliffe Medical Press, Oxford.

- White R and Attwood M (eds) (2000) *Professional Development: A guide for general practice.* Blackwells, Oxford.

- RCGP (2000) *Practice and Personal Development Planning: A tool kit for practices.* North of England Faculty of RCGP, London.

- Grant J, Chambers E and Jackson G (eds) (1999) *The Good CPD Guide: A practical guide to managed CPD.* Open University Centre for Education in Medicine, Reed Business Information.

- Pendleton D and Hasler J (1997) *Professional Development in General Practice.* Oxford University Press, Oxford.

- Robinson L, Story R and Spencer J (1995) Using facilitated discussion for significant event auditing. *BMJ.* **311**: 315–18.

On quality in general practice

- Irvine S and Haman H (2001) *Spotlight on General Practice: Preparing for the demands of clinical governance and revalidation.* Radcliffe Medical Press, Oxford.

- Irvine D and Irvine S (1996) *The Practice of Quality.* Radcliffe Medical Press, Oxford. Out of print.

- Birch K, Field S and Scrivens E (2000) *Quality in General Practice.* Radcliffe Medical Press, Oxford.

On patient involvement

- Chambers R (2000) *Involving Patients and the Public: How to do it better.* Radcliffe Medical Press, Oxford.

- DoH (1998) *In the Public Interest: Developing a strategy for public participation in the NHS.* Department of Health, London.

On stress management

- Chambers R (1999) *Survival Skills for General Practitioners.* Radcliffe Medical Press, Oxford.
- Chambers R and Davies M (1999) *What Stress.* RCGP, London.
- Haslam D (ed.) (2000) *Not Another Guide to Stress in General Practice!* (2e). Radcliffe Medical Press, Oxford.

Training and development sources

Sources of appraisal information

Consultation Satisfaction Questionnaire in booklet or disk form at £5 each from:

National Centre for Clinical Audit
Department of General Practice
Gwendolen Road
Leicester LE5 4PE
Tel: 0116 258 4871

PUNs and DENs – copies of log book, with worked examples, for £3.00 + p&p from:

Dr Richard Eve
Lime Tree
Mount Street
Bishop Lydeard
Taunton TA4 3LH
Tel: 01823 432089
Fax: 01823 326755

email: eve97@msn.com

MCQ tests from:

RCGP (Scotland)
25 Queen Street
Edinburgh EH2 1JX
Tel: 0131 260 6800
Fax: 0131 260 6836

email: scottish@rcgp.org.uk

Insight 360° – a computer-based tool for practice team feedback in appraisal, available from:

Edgecumbe Consulting
125 Pembroke Road
Clifton
Bristol BS8 3ES
Tel: 0117 973 8899
Fax: 0117 973 8844

email: consulting@edgecumbe.co.uk

Rating Scales – the Northumbria Vocational Training Scheme Rating Scale and Staff Assessment Questionnaire are available from:

North Northumberland Trainer Group
www.wcsquare.demon.co.uk

or

The Postgraduate Institute for Medicine and Dentistry
10–12 Framlington Place
Newcastle upon Tyne NE2 4AB
Tel: 0191 222 7029
Fax: 0191 221 1049

www.ncl.ac.uk/pimd

Facilitation

Help and local advice should be sought from your local postgraduate institution, or health authority, or from Hilary Haman or Sally Irvine.

Haman and Irvine Associates
Tel: 01670 517546 or 02920 569220
Fax: 01670 510046 or 02920 575959

email: hiaconsultants@hotmail.com

Index